CARING FOR YOUR UNBORN CHILD

CARING FOR YOUR UNBORN CHILD

HOW TO GIVE YOUR BABY THE BEST POSSIBLE START IN LIFE

Roy Ridgway

THORSONS

Thorsons Publishing Group

First published in 1990

For Michaela, Mary Ann,
Lawrence and Katie

Illustrations by Jane Bowden

British Library Cataloguing in Publication Data

Ridgway, Roy
Caring for your unborn child.
1. Women. Pregnancy. Health matters
I. Title
618.24

ISBN 0-7225-1740-8

Published by Thorsons Publishers Limited, Wellingborough, Northamptonshire

Typeset by Harper Phototypesetters Limited, Northampton, England

Printed in Great Britain by
Woolnough Bookbinding Ltd, Irthlingborough, Northamptonshire

1 3 5 7 9 10 8 6 4 2

Contents

Author's Note:
Throughout the book, apart from the opening paragraph, I have adopted the convention of using 'he' (referring to young children, including the unborn child) to mean 'he or she'. I am aware of objections to this, but where a book is centrally concerned with interaction between mother and child, it is far less confusing to adopt this convention.

Introduction

This is not a book about a medical condition. It's not about pregnancy and it's not about the foetus. The foetus is a word invented by doctors to describe a witless creature who gives its host, the mother, a lot of discomfort and anguish and who needs a lot of medical attention. This is not, in fact, a medical book, though there is some reference to illness. The illness, however, is mainly in the environment. Clear that up and a lot of the diseases of mankind – and womankind – will disappear! What I am writing about in this book is the wonderful and dramatic beginning of human life; the struggle of a human being to adapt and grow and to communicate his or her needs to the outside world, a world which either doesn't believe he is human or largely ignores him. So, unlike many other books about pregnancy, the main actor in this scenario is the unborn child. The main supporting cast are the parents, of course, with a number of others standing in the wings, waiting to come on, such as the obstetrician or midwife and sundry relatives, who are there to help when they can, and are expected to do as they're told and not to try to run the show.

My thanks are due to many people, too numerous to mention here, who have helped me in various ways to put this book together, but mainly to my colleagues in the International Society for Prenatal and Perinatal Psychology and Medicine, who have provided many of the ideas for it. In particular, I should like to thank Eve Bowen, Dr David Chamberlain, Dr Rene Van de Carr, and Dr Brent Logan for providing me with a great deal of fascinating material, from which I have quoted. I would also like to thank my wife, Dorothea, for all the research work she has done on my behalf and for putting up with my swings of mood (like an expectant father's) while working on this book, which is *my* baby, who has arrived a bit late in my life. I wish I'd met someone like him a long time ago. However, I hope my 'baby' will be welcomed by couples everywhere and introduce them to a new way of looking at pregnancy and birth and caring for the unborn child.

Roy Ridgway

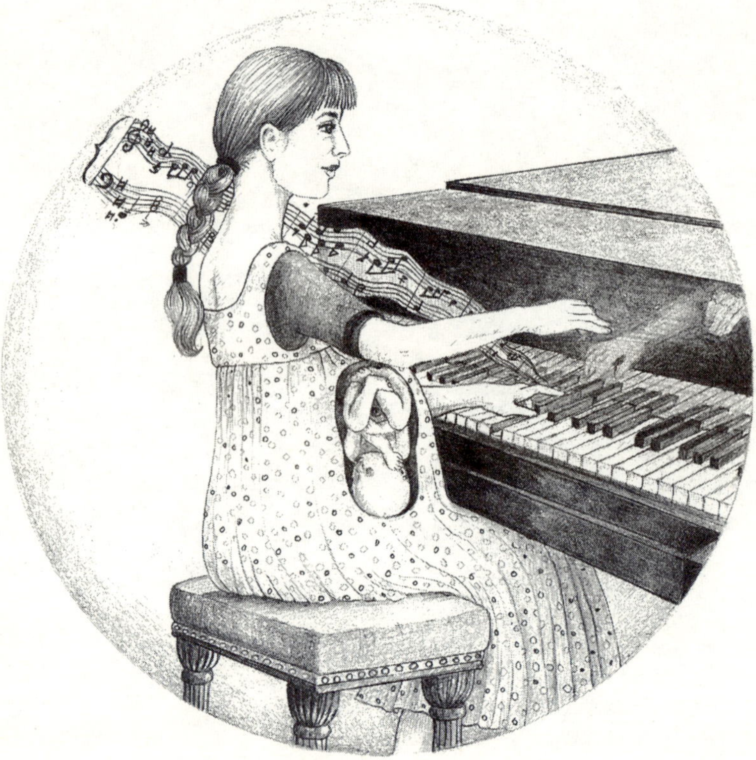

1

Life before birth

What do you say when the doctor or midwife places your newborn baby on your stomach? How do you greet him or her? Do you say anything? Possibly not. This is more a time for squeals and 'Ooh!'s and 'Ah!'s than words, but you will probably ask yourself, 'Who is this little wriggly creature with the screwed-up face? Is he really mine?' Then perhaps you will turn to your partner, standing there at the side of the bed, looking stunned and bewildered, and with a smile that says, 'See, I've done it', you will hastily add, 'He's ours. *Our* child! Can you believe it?'

You will perhaps hold the child up as if he were some kind of trophy awarded to you for a race won: a marathon race that went on and on. And then perhaps you and your partner will go through the ritual of counting fingers and toes to make sure that they are all there.

The child's anatomy will be carefully scrutinized for the slightest blemish. You will regard him first of all as yours, *all* yours: eyes, ears, limbs, the smell of him, the feel of him, the sound of him. You will probably find holding him is a very sensuous experience, but with a difference: it will not be exactly like holding another person. It will feel like holding someone who has sprung from nowhere and is intimately yours, closer to you than anybody you have ever known apart from your own mother when you were a baby. You will look at him with pride. And if, as is likely, you find no flaws, you will feel very pleased with yourself. He's your perfect, flawless work of art.

But it's not long before you begin to wonder who's boss – him or you? And that's when he starts asserting himself. He's a little individual, no longer a part of you. You watch for his responses:

for a hand that moves tentatively to grasp some object, or for the flicker of a smile.

The fact of the matter is that you don't really know your baby or try to get to know him until after he is born. *He* probably knows *you* far better than you know him. He's probably much more confident about himself and where he is than you are. As far as he is concerned, he's been around a long time and has acquired a number of skills in the womb, which he puts to very good use within a few hours of birth.

He's been listening to you and getting to know you for some time before he has become visible to you. Yes, he *really* knows you. But not as someone separate. You are his world – his entire world.

Within a few moments of birth a baby can communicate with his mother. He can recognize her voice, which he's got to know very well. His hearing in the womb is extraordinarily acute. In the womb during the weeks before birth he can hear all kinds of sounds, some of them so high or low that they cannot be heard by the adult ear. He can even distinguish between various sounds of words or notes of music. He is calmed by a lullaby, but maddened by any sudden loud noise. He quite likes the sound of the mother's heart beat, of course, or even her stomach rumblings, which peak at a surprising 85 to 90 decibels, but he jumps when he hears a car backfire or a door slam. He's even been known to object to the sound of a typewriter. There was, in fact, a typist who was forced to give up her job during her eighth month of pregnancy because every time the typewriter carriage was returned to begin a new line, the clang caused the unborn baby to jump. With 30 lines to a page, the typist just couldn't take all that jumping.

The psychotherapist Arthur Janov, of Primal Scream fame, wrote about a mother who reported that, when she was eight months pregnant, she went to a park which had a rifle range. Each time a shot was fired, said the woman, she felt her baby jump in the abdomen. When the baby was eight months old, she returned to the same park; and when a shot was fired, the baby had a startled reaction, more extreme than might be expected, according to her mother.

Instinctively, the mother can recognize her own baby's voice – the gurgles and cries – and can usually distinguish it from another baby's. And, if she trusts her own instinct, she usually knows what the cries mean. She knows if the baby is hungry or tired or if his nappy is wet. There's communication right from the start, from the moment of birth.

A mother, of course, has to get used to having a baby making demands. But she doesn't mind. She loves it. Her partner, however, is a little more apprehensive, not quite so enraptured, mainly because he hasn't lived so closely to the baby as the mother, who, for months has been aware of the baby's life growing and throbbing inside her. Her body has been responding all the time to the needs of the developing child. For her partner, it's a bit different. He's been on the outside, so to speak, not sharing in the development of the new life. Apart from the thrill of feeling the kicks at what is known as the 'quickening' – a misnomer because the baby kicks long before he makes his presence felt – he usually experiences the baby for the first time at the moment of birth.

Unprepared for the baby

There are some parents who are totally unprepared for childbirth. They have no idea what to expect. Take, for instance, Mrs V.:

'I remember when he was first born. I just couldn't see him as my baby. He was a stranger. I hadn't really imagined what he would look like or anything about him when he was unborn, so I was really surprised . . .'

Mrs V., who panicked when her baby was born, was an adolescent and had dropped out of school and married someone slightly younger than herself. The young couple decided to have a child, but didn't think about it very much. Mrs V. just stopped taking the Pill. 'Why not have a child?' Mrs V. said. 'It was sort of crazy . . . I was tired of my birth control pills just then.'

Not all couples are as casual about having a baby as Mrs V. and her young husband, whose story is told by Judith Ballou, a clinical psychologist at the University of Michigan's Medical Center, in her book *The Psychology of Pregnancy.*

Many couples, however, though aware of their responsibility, do not appreciate what an impact the child is going to make on their lives. They talk about the child, of course. The mother will say things like 'Will I be able to cope? Will the child be too demanding? What's going to happen to me?'

A mother is often ambivalent about the child. She may not be absolutely sure she wants a baby. She has moods like that when she hates the whole business of pregnancy, though she probably keeps such thoughts to herself. There are also those fears, not usually expressed, that the child may be abnormal. 'Will it have all its arms and legs?'

Most couples will hardly be aware of the child's existence as a separate person before his kicking is felt – unless, that is, they know about the need for preconceptual care. A child's life does not begin at conception, but before: psychologically, with the parents' expectations, and physically, with their state of health. Therefore it is important that before deciding to have a baby, the couple should learn something about the way a child, a human being, begins life, and about what his needs are *before* conception. You are very careful about what you give a child to eat and about how much sleep he should have once he is born. You are also careful about your own health during pregnancy because you are aware that you need to be well to nourish the child in your womb. But you may not consider it necessary to prepare yourself for conception.

The child's health depends, to a great extent, on your health and your partner's health before conception. The man's health is just as important as the woman's. In fact, many birth defects are caused by the poor quality of the man's sperm.

Then, after conception, you should know what the child's needs are in the womb. Things can go drastically wrong if the conditions for the child's health as he develops in the womb are not met, particularly in the early stages of pregnancy.

Life in the womb

Our knowledge of life in the womb is expanding all the time. With our modern scanners we can chart the growth of the unborn baby, monitor its every move: its heartbeat, its hand and leg movements, its reactions to stimulation of various kinds, including toxins such as alcohol or nicotine. Health checks can be made, blood samples taken, and the child in the womb can be treated for a variety of conditions, such as low weight or anaemia.

We know every step of the child's development in the womb from the moment of conception when the male sperm fuses with a female ovum. Fertilization is followed by the doubling-up of cells, which goes on throughout pregnancy. Forty-five generations of this doubling-up of cells are needed to reach the thirty million million of the mature adult. Forty-one of the forty-five divisions take place before birth.

'From the point of view of the sort of person we are going to be', said the New Zealand gynaecologist, Professor A. M. Liley, '90 per cent of the excitement is over by the time we are born.'

Professor Liley wasn't the first to recognize that the events in the womb were, from the point of view of the child's personality and health, of more importance than anything that followed. The poet Samuel Taylor Coleridge said something similar in 1802. He had read Thomas Browne's observation that we were some months older than we said we were, because we had lived, moved, and had our being in that other world, our mother's womb. 'Yes,' said Coleridge, 'the history of man for the nine months preceding birth would probably be far more interesting and contain events of greater moment than all the threescore and ten that follow it.'

The early days and weeks of pregnancy are the most hazardous. That is the time when the unborn child is at its most vulnerable, when the mother may not even know she is pregnant and may be smoking and drinking and eating all the wrong kinds of food, all of which could put her child at risk or damage it irreversibly. 'That is why', said Liley, 'we regard the care of the pregnant woman, and this early stage of life, as so important. If anything goes wrong then, it can cast its shadow far into the future.'

Four days after conception, about 32 cells form a hollow ball called the blastocyst; and from then until implantation is a pretty treacherous obstacle course for this tiny human being. There is a person there – a life seeking to establish itself. That life moves and splutters in those first cells and will go on vibrating throughout pregnancy until it manifests itself in the first cries of the newborn baby. That moment when the baby is born is the end of a long trail.

It felt safe and secure in the womb, but it's touch and go during the first few days. That bundle of cells, the blastocyst, grows finger-like projections (called the chorionic villi) which cling on to the lining of the uterus (the endometrium) for dear life! At first the uterus reacts to the blastocyst as if it were an invading intruder. The lining tissues swell to engulf the embryo and at the same time, thousands of white blood cells are marshalled to get rid of any debris. It really is a bloody battle. That tiny blastocyst, fighting for its life, has no more than a 50-50 chance of surviving.

Struggle for survival

There are many who say that this struggle for survival in the womb becomes a part of our 'cellular' memory, buried deep in the unconscious, which serves as a template for postnatal behaviour. Everything that has happened to us, from the very beginning, is recorded somewhere deep within ourselves and influences our behaviour. We may not be able to retrieve these memories, but nothing is lost. It is our memories, in fact, which hold us together. We can only remain upright because we *learned* to walk; and the memory of each step we took, and the way we were able to maintain our balance, has been incorporated into our way of behaviour – into the totality of our actions. Each person learns in a slightly different way. Each person has his own style.

There are memories of growth, of obstacles encountered, victories won: memories of everything that has ever taken place, physically and emotionally. 'There's a memory of the body,' said psychologist Otto Rank, 'a visceral memory in the blood, in the muscles.'

I shall be discussing this later. I only mention it here because there is growing evidence that whatever happens to us in the womb will influence us, not only because of the physical conditions, which could perhaps lead to ill-health, but because of parental attitudes, fears, anxieties, and so on. The emotional environment is as important as the physical. In fact, the two cannot be separated. They interact. So when we talk about the unborn child we are not talking about some passive, witless creature which has been given the medical term 'foetus': we are talking about a real child, a human being. And in this book we are talking about caring for that human being during the whole course of his life in the womb. If we focus our attention on the child we shall also be doing what's best for the mother, because the child is going to insist throughout pregnancy on being cared for, and if the mother ignores the child, she is going to suffer.

Therefore, I suggest that an expectant mother should see herself not just as pregnant but throughout those nine months – and not just after the child becomes visible at birth – as a mother caring for her child, protecting and nourishing him. She'd do this after birth, so why not before birth? He's the same person. And, of course, *both* parents must become involved. They must both accept the responsibility of caring for their unborn child.

Life begins at conception

Here, I should like to repeat something I wrote in a previous book, *The Unborn Child: How to recognise and overcome prenatal trauma* (1987) in which I compared humanistic psychology, and how it defines the human being, with modern embryology and how it describes the early development of human life. Humanistic psychology, and especially the psychology of its founder, Abraham Maslow – who described it as 'the science of Being' – is based on the assumption that a person's deepest need is to be fully human, to realize his full potential, which means becoming the person he truly is. From the start he has an essential inner nature, which is in part unique and in part species-wide.

This fits the facts of modern embryology. For instance, the embryologist Erich Blechschmidt maintains that development in the womb is about preserving what is there at the start. In other words, at the moment of conception there's an individual life, which is best preserved by the way the body grows – tissues, muscles, nerves, bones, organs – in the womb. The function of each step in the development of the embryo, and later the foetus, is to maintain a balance between all the parts of the body, and to adapt to the conditions in the womb. It's a reactive process. You could describe this process as the body protecting the spirit, or the outside protecting the inside.

Each stage of development is an adaptation to external changes in accordance with genetically coded instructions. Blechschmidt describes growth as the operation of two complementary forces – those of heredity and of adaptation. 'Without the cellular membrane there would be no food intake and, consequently, no growth; without the nucleus (which carries the genetic code) there would be no heredity influence in propagation.'

The operation of these forces, one coming from inside and the other from outside, sounds like the yin and yang of Taoism: the 'firm' and assertive (yin) establishing a direction according to the genetic code; and the 'yielding' or accepting (yang) allowing the penetration by a benign force that provides nourishment for growth.

To me the most staggering fact about human existence is the fact, confirmed by modern embryology, that each one of us has a unique inner nature that is there from conception to death, struggling all the time to assert itself. How many times have you heard someone say, 'I can't make myself heard', or, 'I'm not allowed to be myself'? That's the real you, an expression of the frustration you feel within yourself. It's the real you (not your self-image, which is the result of social conditioning) that was there at the start, and may have been smothered at birth and is crying out for recognition: a sad story, and one that starts with parents' expectations at the moment they are told a child is on the way. That is the moment when an individual life begins. It begins with a feeling, an inner feeling which never leaves you, which is what life is. As Keats wrote, 'Life is the rose's hope while yet unblown' – the flower that is there before it becomes visible. Life is a feeling at the heart of one's being – sometimes described as pure subjectivity – that is blocked later by the psychological needs of others, and, inter-linked with this, your own psychological fears.

Ashley Montagu, in *Life Before Birth,* (New American Library, 1961), puts it like this:

> The basic fact is simple: life begins, not at birth, but at conception.
>
> This means that a developing child is alive not only in the sense that he is composed of living tissues, but also in the sense that from the moment of conception *things happen to him.* Furthermore, when things happen to him, even though he may be only two weeks old (in the womb), and he looks more like a creature from another world than a potential human being, and his birth date is eight and a half months in the future, he reacts. In spite of his newness and his appearance, he is a living, striving organism from the very beginning.

That's absolutely right, except for the use of the words 'potential' and 'organism'. He *is* a human being from the very beginning: your child.

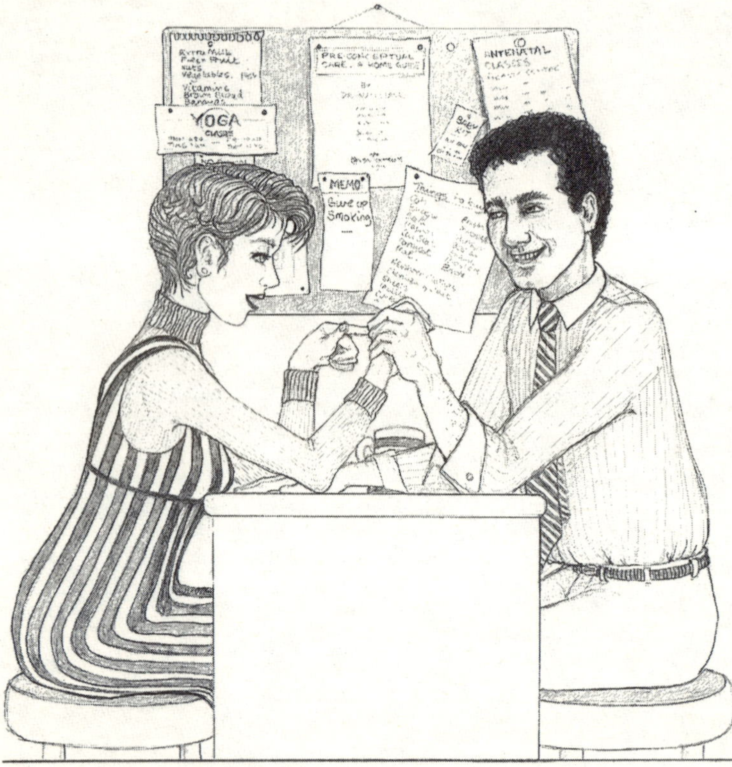
Extra Milk
Fresh Fruit
nuts
Vegetables. Fish
Vitamins
Brown Bread
Bananas
YOGA
CLASSES
PRE-CONCEPTUAL CARE. A HOME GUIDE
ANTENATAL
CLASSES
MEMO
Give up Smoking

2

Preparing to have a child

You make careful preparations for all sorts of events in your life, some important, like a wedding, or some quite trivial, like what you're going to have for dinner, but many couples make no preparations at all for what is perhaps the most important event of all, the conception of a human life. For many, pregnancy just happens. It's not planned with the same care as other important life events.

It's not that couples are indifferent about starting a family. The majority of them are delighted when they discover that a child is on the way. Then their lives do change and they will do all they can to avoid any possible risk to the child. But what is not generally appreciated is that when a woman discovers she is pregnant, if she is not living a healthy lifestyle at the moment of conception and in the weeks that follow, the health of her child may already have been put at risk. If she smokes or drinks, for instance, she could have damaged her child before she even knows she is pregnant. And it's not only the mother's health that is important: the father too can damage the child because of the poor quality of his sperm, caused by smoking and/or the consumption of alcohol.

The argument against preconceptual care is that it puts an extra burden on the woman, making her feel guilty if her child is not as healthy as she'd hoped. She blames herself for anything that may go wrong after birth. It's true that mothers in the past have been loaded with an enormous responsibility for the rearing of their children; and the mother of today, who goes out to work, and may be ambitious about succeeding in her chosen career, may be made to feel that she has neglected her children.

This is all wrong. First of all, a successful pregnancy and the health of the child are the responsibility of both parents. But educating for all that is involved in pregnancy, including pre-pregnancy health, is also society's responsibility. Preconceptual care should be taught in our schools. There should be courses on preconceptual care at our further education establishments. In fact, as much attention should be paid to preparing a couple for pregnancy as antenatal care during pregnancy.

The child's health depends to a large extent on the mental and physical health of the couple at the moment of conception. It is not true, as many people imagine, that most pregnancies are normal. It depends, of course, on what you mean by normal. Most of us would say that it is quite normal for a child to come kicking and screaming into the world.

At the Prelearning Institute in Snohomish, Washington, USA, they don't, in fact, believe this is normal. Dr Brent Logan, who is director of the Institute, where they teach 'pre-learning' of an unborn child, describes what he regards as a normal, healthy delivery:

> As deliveries go, it was a dream: birth on the due date, short labour, no complications — despite a 10 pound, 7 ounce boy, 20½ inches long, 14½ inches head circumference . . . from an averaged-sized mother. But what additionally delighted family and hospital staff was the child himself: Edward had emerged with eyes wide, smiling, body relaxed, hands open, arms outstretched, and no crying whatsoever; moreover, upon encountering his new universe, he immediately and clearly called 'Mama, Mama, Mama!'

You find this difficult to believe? Well, so did the obstetrician and nurse who delivered the child. This was quite a new experience for them.

Greeting his son from across the room, Edward's father beamed when the infant turned directly to him, staring for a full half-minute. The gynaecologist's professional assessment of the child was: 'Extremely calm, attentive, alert, and healthy.'

This was not an exceptional delivery. In a pilot study, evaluating a new method of prenatal stimulation (which I shall be discussing in chapter 7) there were eight other children born with the same abilities, who were just as attentive, calm and healthy.

It may come as a surprise to some that a normal, healthy child is born with many skills, more than have been recognized in the past, which he has acquired before birth. The child can work out what is going on around him, make choices, signal approval or disapproval. He is not the helpless creature he was once supposed to be, with a brain that is empty and needs to be trained to think, look, perceive, discriminate between people, between objects, sounds, tastes, distances. He can do all these things soon after he is born without any further training: it's all happened in the womb.

There have been many studies of what the American paediatrician Dr M. H. Klaus calls 'the amazing newborn'. Among them have been the studies of that most persistent and critical of baby-watchers, Professor Tom Bower of Edinburgh University, who has shown that a baby is born with certain intellectual skills which no one once thought was possible.

But all this can be put in jeopardy by the parents' lifestyle before conception. There can be neurological damage in the very early stage of embryonic development when the neural tube – the central nervous system – is developing.

Countdown to pregnancy

For the sake of your unborn child you should start a programme of getting fit to have a child six months before becoming pregnant. The following are the most important steps you should take:

1. *Smoking.* A doctor will tell you that the single most damaging thing you can do to your own health and the health of your unborn child is to smoke. If you are planning to start a family, you and your partner should give up smoking six months before pregnancy. This is the first step in your countdown to pregnancy; the first step because, if you are a heavy smoker, it will probably be the most difficult thing you will have to do.

Smoking is a major cause of physical abnormalities and avoidable ill-health in the unborn child. The toxins in tobacco smoke can damage the developing embryo, when rapidly-growing cells are at their most vulnerable, and that may mean before you even know you are pregnant. The risks include miscarriages and stillbirths; damage to the placenta – which is the unborn child's life-support system – due probably to a decreased supply of oxygen; and low birth weight.

In the man, smoking is one of the factors involved in a lowering of the sperm count, which is associated with a toxic condition. It is believed that as many as 80 per cent of birth defects are attributable to the male parent. Besides smoking, other factors involved in damaging sperm include alcohol consumption, poor diet, and environmental pollutants. Apart from the damage to his own health, a man who smokes while his partner is pregnant can damage the health of the unborn child through polluting the home environment, and can cause asthma in the newborn.

As a British Medical Association leaflet says, 'You owe it to yourselves, your family and your future not to smoke.'

2. *Alcohol.* The second step is to cut down on alcohol. It is important to get your alcohol consumption down before conception because damage from alcohol can occur during the course of the monthly cycle, just before the egg leaves the ovum, when the chromosomes become active in preparation for possible fusion with the sperm.

There are 800 clinical and research papers describing the ill-effects of alcohol on the unborn child. Dr Ann Striessguth, a researcher at the University of Washington, USA, listed the main risks to the unborn child as mental retardation; retarded growth; damage to the central nervous system; a variety of other malformations; and death of the unborn child in the womb.

Recent research suggests that it can do no harm to drink below ten units of alcohol a week, a unit being half a pint of ordinary beer or lager; one standard measure of spirits; one standard glass of wine; or one standard small measure of sherry. But it would be wiser to cut out all alcohol during pregnancy. The ill-effects of alcohol on women are more severe than on men, because women's bodies are usually smaller and tend to have a higher proportion of fat to water, which means alcohol is more concentrated in the body fluids.

If you have a serious alcohol problem, you should seek professional advice or counselling long before you decide to start a family.

3. *Diet.* The third step is to pay more attention to your diet,

especially if you are in the habit of eating convenience foods and going to work, as many couples do, without much in the way of breakfast. You should start eating for health, as much for the sake of your child as for yourself. This doesn't mean that your diet must be boring. As a matter of fact, the kind of diet that is good for you is one that has been enjoyed for centuries by families: dairy products, meat, fish, fruit and vegetables.

There are, however, certain foods that we now know could be harmful if indulged in too often. Foods with a high fat content, such as sausages or other fried food, should be eaten as an occasional indulgence and not as a part of your regular diet. Likewise too many eggs, too much high-fat cheese, and too much butter should be avoided. Butter should be replaced, except on special occasions, by polyunsaturated margarines, and if you do use a lot of milk, avoid creamy milk except occasionally in tea or coffee. Use skimmed milk for cooking and for breakfast cereals. But remember, I am talking here about the run-up to pregnancy. You may have to increase your intake of some of these foods – cheese and eggs, for instance – during pregnancy because you'll need extra energy to cope with the increased activity in your body.

Fats (technically known as *lipids*) are needed to provide energy, but it is now believed that high levels of fat in the blood can cause a condition known as *atheroma,* in which fatty plaques build up on the artery walls. The plaques combined with blood can block the arteries and cause heart attacks and strokes.

Nowadays we are becoming much more diet conscious and most people are aware of the value of high-fibre food. But don't go mad about this. You need a certain amount of fibre (which we used to call roughage) but you don't have to go on eating it all the time. Other forms of food, such as the protein to be found in fish, for instance, are just as necessary. But it's a good idea to avoid refined food from which many of the nutrients have been extracted. The food you find on the shelves of the supermarket, which you buy because they can be 'cooked in a jiffy', should be avoided. Eat plenty of fruit and vegetables, but wash them well before eating or cooking to remove residues of pesticides on the skins.

There are a number of excellent books on the market dealing with diet and containing mouth-watering recipes. Barbara

Pickard's *Eating Well for a Healthy Pregnancy* (Sheldon Press, London, 1984) can be recommended. It is a very useful guide to healthy eating before, and after pregnancy. My own book *Preparing for Parenthood* (Penguin, 1990) contains more detailed information on the balanced sort of diet to aim for before pregnancy.

4. *Exercise.* In Western urban society hardly anyone gets all the exercise they need to keep their limbs and spine supple, their muscles strong, and their lungs functioning efficiently. Every day we spend hours travelling in cars and trains and planes, and do an awful lot of sitting. Our bodies were designed principally for movement, not for sitting. Exercise is an important part of health and during the six months' countdown to pregnancy a couple should do all the exercising they can. Stop taking the car to the shops and sitting slouched in a chair watching television for hours on end! If you have an office job, you should get up and move about and, if possible, do something energetic at least once an hour. This is not only good for the body but will improve your performance at most desk jobs. It improves lung function, and therefore increases oxygen uptake in the body and brain. It wakes you up. And it also lowers blood pressure, and provides more energy and the ability to keep going for long periods of activity.

One of the main objects of exercising for pregnancy is to prevent all those aches and pains that occur as the baby grows in the womb and presses down on the pelvis, upsetting the body's natural balance. Exercises to improve your posture are well worth while before pregnancy. You will later find it easier to adjust to the changes that occur in the body.

Alexander Technique

The Alexander Technique is the best way of improving posture. It is not so much an exercise as a way of living – a way of getting rid of bad habits and of restoring the body to its natural way of moving. It is mainly a matter of making you aware of what you are doing wrong. F. M. Alexander, the Australian who invented the technique, said, 'When you stop doing the wrong thing, the right thing does itself.'

It is best to learn the technique from an experienced teacher because there are many individual differences in body posture. By using his hands a teacher can show you what you need to do to correct bad habits in the way you sit, stand, walk or lie down. You need to know about what Alexander calls 'inhibiting' unwanted movements or stresses in the body.

Yoga

Yoga exercises are also excellent as a preparation for pregnancy. So many exercises are painful and leave you tired and discouraged, but not so yoga – if it is practised correctly. In every exercise or posture (asana) the important thing is the quality of movement rather than the effort you put into it. In classical yoga, mind, body and spirit are involved in every exercise. In fact yoga, as it is practised in the East, is a spiritual discipline aiming at achieving harmony between body and spirit.

Again, it is best to learn the exercises from an experienced teacher. There are exercises for individual needs, including some that will help you when your baby starts to grow in the womb and your balance is altered. Yoga breathing is also very helpful. Much of our breathing is haphazard and there are those who say that our breathing went wrong at the start of our lives at the moment of birth. Leonard Orr, for instance, who practises a technique called healing the breath, says that we learned to breathe in the middle of pain and for this reason breathing is associated with fear, so we have never learned to breathe fully and efficiently. Through holding back we create tensions in the body. Be that as it may, the fact is that many of us breathe mostly from the chest and not, as we should, from the stomach. In yoga you are taught 'complete breathing'. You experience wave-like movements as the diaphragm moves up and down and the ribcage expands and contracts as you breathe in and out. It is experienced as one uniform movement. Breathing is important for the expectant mother. Control of breathing, for instance, will help you during the contractions of childbirth.

If you find yoga breathing exercises too difficult, swimming is an excellent way of achieving control over your breathing.

Whatever you do, it is not a good idea to exercise too vigorously. According to Judith Lumley, a senior lecturer in the Department of Obstetrics and Gynaecology at Monash University, Melbourne, strenuous exercise can cause infertility or reduce birth weight in your baby, besides damaging joints and ligaments. You should walk rather than jog. When walking, the force of the body on the knees and hips is one-and-a-half times your body weight and on the ankles two-and-a-half times your weight. When you jog, this force is much greater and there is a risk of damaging weak muscles in the legs.

Psychological effects of bodily rhythms on the unborn child

So far we have emphasized the importance of getting fit for pregnancy from the point of view of the physical health of the mother and child. What is not generally appreciated is the fact that the mother's general sense of well-being, her biological rhythms, and her general functioning could have an important psychological effect on the development of the unborn child.

The growing child in the womb is cradled in an environment of bodily sounds and movements. The way the mother holds herself and the way she moves are important in the development of the unborn child's sense of a pattern of movement that is reassuring if it is regular and rhythmical, but could be disturbing if it is irregular and jerky. Any sudden jerky movement, for instance, will make the child kick in protest, when, in the later stage of pregnancy, his movements begin to be felt.

The importance of rhythmical movement in giving a child a sense of security has long been recognized. A mother will rock her baby to sleep. This gentle rocking movement recalls the movement that the child experienced in the womb. The pattern of movement in the womb, which was imposed on the unborn child's musculature, and then on the brain itself, is imprinted on the body's memory and remains like a permanent motion picture that influences his consciousness and subsequent reactions. Even in ancient Greece the importance of movement was recognized. Plato, in *The Laws* (Book VII) wrote:

> So let's take this as our basic principle . . . all young children, and especially very tiny infants, benefit both physically and mentally from being nursed and kept in motion, as far as practicable, throughout the day and night; indeed, if only it could be managed, they ought to live as though they were permanently on board ship. But as that's impossible, we must aim to provide our new-born infants with the closest possible approximation to this ideal.

The rhythms, both of sound and movement, that we all find so pleasurable, were first established in the womb. They remain with us as memory traces. So, from this point of view, it could be important for a prospective mother to try to establish good habits of posture and movement; and the best time to begin a programme of exercises, such as those described above, is before pregnancy.

Relationships

Like any other important life event, pregnancy doesn't only affect the person experiencing it, but it is also likely to have a profound and complex effect on a whole network of relationships extending beyond the couple who are most affected. In the first place, the pregnant woman has to adjust to the image of the child within herself – the love object who at first is perceived as part of the self; and then as the child grows in the womb and he becomes visible on a scanner, he is perceived as existing outside the self as a separate person.

This separate person becomes a central figure in a web of relationships. All the family, including the extended family, are drawn towards him; and everyone has something to say about him. A sibling may be jealous or may think of the unborn child as a future playmate. A husband may feel excluded. In-laws may be delighted and full of concern for the mother. There are all kinds of undercurrents, hopes, fears and jealousies going on that will change the pattern of relationships within the family.

Grete Bibring, a psychoanalyst who studied the psychological processes of pregnancy, sums up the feelings of a woman who is pregnant for the first time by telling the story of a girl who arrived at an antenatal clinic in an agitated state and started to talk as she stood in the doorway. Bibring reports her as saying: 'I was terribly excited and anxious last night. I suddenly realized that I won't be Jenny much longer, but Mother for ever and ever after.' She went on to talk, more calmly, about her own mother. She said she was pleased when she left home and became independent. After that she rarely visited her mother. But she said that 'last night' she had realized that whenever she had some terrible problem, her first thought had always been, what would her mother say? And this, she felt, would be her role in the life of her own child. She would become her child's guide and confidante. Her relationship with her own mother would then change: she would become more of an equal.

Bibring says that, when a woman becomes pregnant, running like a thread through all her relationships is her relationship with her own mother. It is usually the mother that provides the prototype of a parental figure. This can be reassuring to the pregnant woman, but it can also create tensions between her and her husband and her husband's family.

It is only in recent years that the father's role in pregnancy has been fully recognized. There was a time when the father was regarded almost as if he was an outsider. The midwife felt that it was best for him to be well out of the way. This is still the case in the Soviet Union, where the father is not even allowed in the hospital, for fear that he will bring in some infection from outside. He must wait until mother and child go home before seeing the baby.*

Now in the UK and USA more than 80 per cent of fathers see their babies born. Brian Jackson describes in his book *Fatherhood* (Allen and Unwin, 1984), how he felt when he saw his own child born. It was, he said, 'a personal Everest'. Many fathers now share in a very intimate way the miracle of birth; they also have powerful feelings, or rather they don't mind acknowledging powerful feelings any more, during the nine months of pregnancy.

However, there are many couples who don't know what to expect during pregnancy. Their own relationship is of crucial importance; so it is best to get that right before they start a family. For the sake of the child, adjustments will have to be made; there must be complete understanding of what a child means to them both and how they see their responsibilities as parents.

* According to Wendy Savage, a senior lecturer in obstetrics and gynaecology, there is evidence that 'birth perestroika' has begun in Russia. (Letter *Observer,* 11 June, 1989). In an experiment in Riga, husbands were allowed to accompany their pregnant wives into hospital and it was found that the rate of infection did not rise. Following this, a directive was issued by the Soviet Ministry of Health permitting husbands to visit their wives in hospital. A group of British obstetricians and gynaecologists took part in a tour of the Soviet Union in May 1989, under the auspices of the UK-USSR Medical Exchange Programme. The British group was welcomed by Soviet doctors and midwives, who expressed an interest in Western approaches to childbirth.

Learning to be good enough parents

Parents' attitudes to pregnancy, to the idea of starting a family, should not be something isolated from their general approach to health and to the many varied problems that life throws up. How do you go about solving your problems? What do you expect from life? Are you an optimist or pessimist, confident or despondent, or neither one thing nor the other? Just a human being who has experienced many ups and downs, but holds on to a certain faith in life, or in a god, and knows about failure, but believes, in the words of Browning, that 'you fall to rise, are baffled to fight better.' Good enough parents are realistic people and though they will do everything possible for the good of their family, they will not expect miracles. Things will go wrong at times. They know that. There is no blueprint for perfection. Our growth, from the moment of conception, depends mainly on the ability or effort made to adapt to a constantly changing environment. That effort, as we encounter the difficulties that come with life's crises, can be exhilarating or depressing. Life is always a struggle, but there is plenty of joy in the struggle. Even in sickness there are many who find a strength that they didn't know they possessed. Paradoxically, their intrinsic health shines through their sickness. It's this inner strength that matters most of all.

The health of parents and of their children depends on what parents expect out of life. If they expect too much, they will probably give up trying when things start to go wrong. It's our thinking – our philosophy or religion – that is important. That is a big influence, in fact the main influence in the way we behave as parents. The health of our planet, in fact, starts with the way we think about and plan our families and the way we treat our children. When we are planning a family we are planning for life, but let's not be too ambitious. We merely chart our course by the stars – we don't ever expect to reach them. Bruno Bettelheim, who is probably the most distinguished of child psychologists, is the author of a book with the title of *A Good Enough Parent* (Alfred Knopf, New York, 1987). He believes that bringing up a child is a matter of responding to each individual child's needs, and helping him or her to develop into the person he or she wishes to be, rather than following any particular set of rules. He insists that parents must never give in to their desire to create the child they would like to have.

There are some beautiful lines by Khalil Gibran, in his book *The Prophet* (Alfred Knopf, New York, 1923), which proffers the same advice:

> Your children are not your children:
> They are the sons and daughters of Life's longing for itself.
> They came through you but not from you.
> And though they are with you yet they belong not to you.
> You may give them your love but not your thoughts,
> For they have their own thoughts.
> You may have their bodies, but not their souls,
> For their souls dwell in the house of tomorrow, which you cannot visit, not even in your dreams.
> You may strive to be like them, but seek not to make them like you.
> For life goes not backward nor tarries with yesterday.

A child's personality is so often created for him by parents, and mostly it is built up of dos and don'ts. This process of moulding a personality starts with your dream children, who may be there in your imagination even before you find a partner. It is part of the process of breaking away from your own parents. Your child will be treated differently, you say to yourself, from the way your parents treated you. You won't repeat their mistakes. On the other hand, after marriage, you may remember some parts of your own childhood with a great deal of pleasure and may wish to recreate the atmosphere and environment you knew for your own child.

The snag is there are two of you each dreaming his or her own dreams. In many marriages there are more rows about children than about almost anything else. So it's best to go into the whole business of bringing up a family, to talk about it honestly, hammer out differences of approach, and come to some understanding about expectations, and know what your reasons are for wanting a family at all, before you start one. It could be disastrous from the word 'go'. But if you've talked it over, and you both share the same feelings about bringing up children, it could be a great joy.

There are a number of reasons why you *shouldn't* have a child and they include the hope that a baby will patch up a failing relationship or because other people, such as your own parents, want you to have one. The best reason for having a child is a gut reason – because both of you love children and you simply must have one of your own!

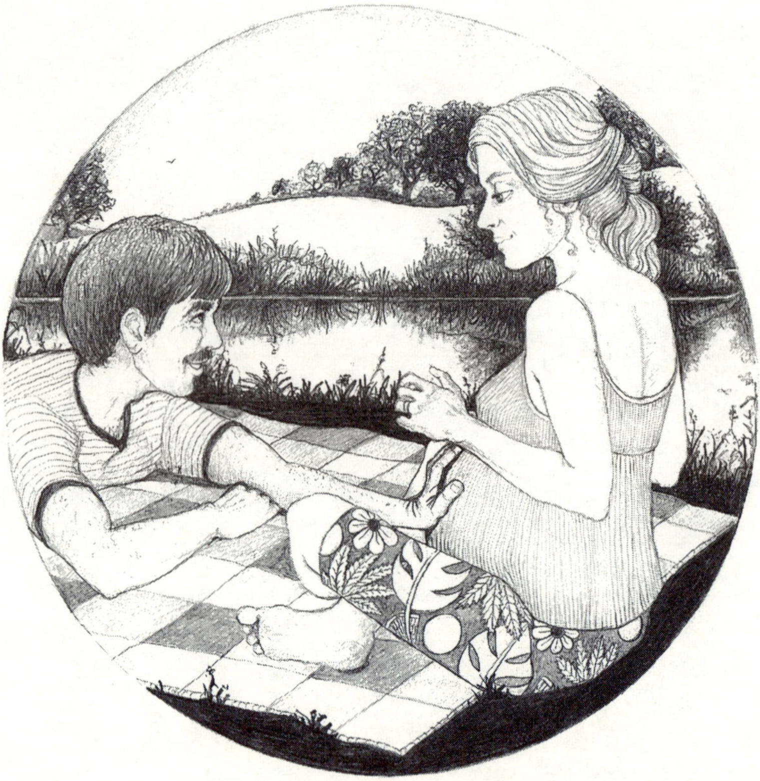

3

The personality of the unborn child

It might seem absurd to some to talk about the foetus as having a personality. For centuries we have regarded the foetus as no more than a person in the making, unable to see or hear or feel anything much, or to respond to stimulation, until after birth. Freud described the state of mind of the unborn child as a condition 'not unlike sleep'. And that great neurophysiologist, Sir Charles Sherrington, spoke of 'the miracle of the human ear developing in silent water for hearing in vibrant ear'. None of this is true.

The moment a child is born a mother will say, 'Oh! he definitely has a personality.' She might describe him as 'stubborn' or 'placid' or 'good-tempered' or 'a little horror!' We have no difficulty in giving a newborn baby a personality. Yet he's no different from the baby who was in the womb only moments before. No doubt some of what we see as 'personality' are our own projections. We *give* him the kind of personality we admire or, if we find a baby difficult to handle, we give him a personality which says more about our own personality problems than his. In this way the personality of a baby begins to be recognizable in a social context; at birth he becomes a social being, interacting with others, being influenced by others. In a sense, he is more truly 'himself' immediately before birth than after.

The egoist

Albert Liley, the New Zealand gynaecologist, was the first to write about the personality of the foetus. In 1972 he chose this title for a scientific paper in the Australian and New Zealand

Psychiatric Journal. His words describing the way the foetus takes control of the mother's pregnancy have often been quoted:

> Far from being an inert passenger in a pregnant mother, the foetus is very much in command of the pregnancy. It is the foetus who guarantees the endocrine success of pregnancy and induces all manner of changes in maternal physiology to make her a suitable host . . . It is the foetus who determines the duration of pregnancy. It is the foetus who decides which way he will be in pregnancy and which way he will present in labour. Even in labour the foetus is not entirely passive – neither the toothpaste in the tube nor the cork in the champagne bottle required by the old hydraulic theories of the mechanics of labour.

In other words, the unborn child is very definitely the boss! The mother must do what he wants her to do. An erring mother, who doesn't provide him with a suitable environment for his development, will suffer.

The British gynaecologist Frank Hytten calls the foetus a little egoist. 'As soon as he has plugged himself into the uterus wall', Dr Hytten says, 'he sets out to make certain that his needs are served, regardless of any inconvenience he may cause.'

This insistence on being cared for and of being provided with all that he needs for his physical and mental development is the main characteristic of the growing child, not only as he develops in the womb, but later when he becomes visible and even more demanding. As Khalil Gibran said in his poem, he does *not* belong to you. He is his own person. So that's the first thing we must recognize about the personality of the unborn child. The essential characteristics of any person, of any human being, are present throughout life from the very beginning until death. T. S. Eliot expressed this in the words: 'In the beginning is our end.'

The here-and-now

It is a common fallacy that all living things are, from the moment of conception, striving towards some goal. We look at the unborn child as incomplete and as if it had some kind of unconscious sense of purpose or direction as it develops to become a fully functioning child. It was once thought that there was a 'centre of organization' consisting of chemical inductors which were responsible for the way the child developed; but no one has ever found any chemical substance that could be responsible for directing the growth of the child. But we still persist in giving the unborn child a sense of direction. And then later, after birth, we look at the child as living mainly for the purpose of becoming an adult.

Some of our cherished beliefs of the past (scientific myths) have been overturned by modern embryology. For instance, embryonic development is not, as some people believe, an evolutionary process in the sense of proceeding from the simple to the complex. At every stage there is a complex set of circumstances that leads to the next stage. The mistake is seeing small as simple and big as complex.

Giving the growing organism in the womb a sense of purpose, says the embryologist Erich Blechschmidt, is 'teleological' thinking, which is unscientific. 'Teleology' is a word derived from the Greek, which simply means a study of ends or goals in relation to the appearance and behaviour patterns of living things; and so 'teleological thinking' means seeing something in terms of what its purpose may be. This way of thinking has influenced almost everything we do for our children. We are always preparing them for what comes next. We keep projecting them into the future. And thus we rob them of their present, which is their childhood. Children are not always allowed to be children, to enjoy themselves in their own way. They must always be doing what parents want or tell them to do 'for their own good'. They must learn to grow up. This is one of the cardinal errors of education: forcing children to become adults, at a pace that is not natural.

The way we see the foetus is influenced by our idea of maturity. This idea, in fact, dominates all our relationships with our fellow human beings and with all living creatures.

Albert Liley points out that medicine is studied by young adults and medical standards of normality are therefore the standards of the young adult – very often male! 'It is part of the arrogance of young adults', says Liley, 'to consider that the only people who matter are young adults.'

Since maturity means adulthood, the foetus is, by definition, regarded as immature, and that, to many people, is the same thing as saying inferior.

Thus, the tendency has developed to consider the foetus, or newborn baby, as a poorly functioning adult rather than as a splendidly functioning baby. 'Every age and stage of life has its excellencies,' Liley says, 'and its weaknesses, and foetal life is no exception. We do not regard the foetal circulatory system, different as it is from the child's or adult's, as one big heap of congenital defects, but rather a system superbly adapted to the circumstances in which it lives.'

The foetus, at every stage of development, is functioning in a particular way that is appropriate. There is nothing there, that anyone can discern, that could be said to be intended for future use. When the child is born there are no useless cells, tissues or organs that have been lying dormant in the womb, waiting for the moment of birth.

All growth in the womb is functional. The hand, for instance, can be seen to develop with a sort of grasping movement. That structure grows in that particular way with that particular function: i.e. to grasp or touch or hold. Every structure as it develops has a function. In fact, you can't separate structure from function: the two go hand in hand. So a need arises which is followed by the satisfaction of that need in the here-and-now. The child is constantly moving in the womb and this movement is associated with growth. As he approaches full term you will see him stretching, kicking, turning somersaults, and, propelled by his feet, moving about to try to make itself comfortable in the womb. He adjusts himself to his mother's posture, until he becomes so big that all movement becomes difficult, and then the child starts the process of birth. 'I'm too big for comfort in this small space,' you can imagine the child saying to himself. 'I must find a way out.' Everything the child does makes sense in the environment of the womb. To the unborn child, that's all there is. There's nothing else: no future state of bliss or fulfilment towards which he is moving.

Another thing, then, that you can say about the personality of the unborn child is that the child is not waiting to be born or waiting to be a human being. He is not concerned with the future; he is only concerned with adjusting to the situation as he finds it from moment to moment. He is truly living and struggling and adapting to his situation in the here-and-now.

You can see from what I have said so far that our attitude to the unborn child is more or less the same as our attitude to the child after birth. He is small and helpless, we say; he is immature; he is not 'all there'; and he belongs to us. And so the child grows up into adulthood feeling that there is always another step ahead, another goal to be attained. And because of this his life can become a misery. In fact, many adults are still children waiting to grow up. So the way we see the unborn child, the way we care for him, can influence the whole of his life.

The Development of Life before Birth

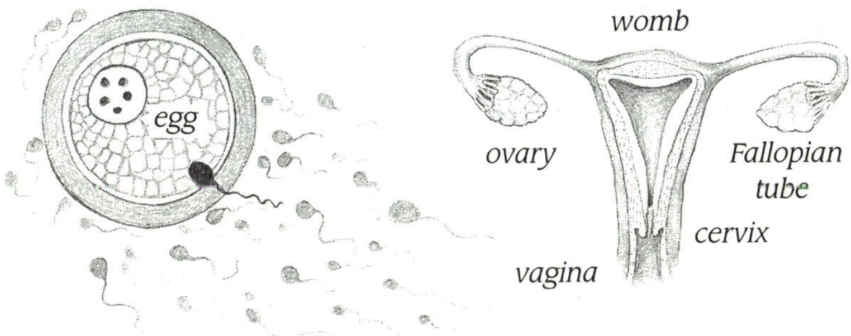

Conception (fertilization)

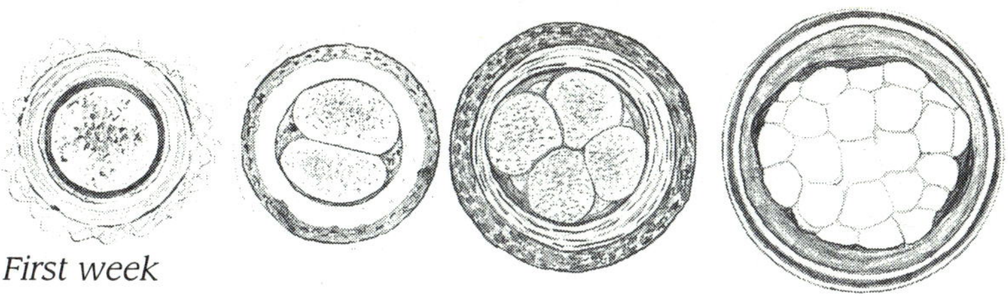

First week

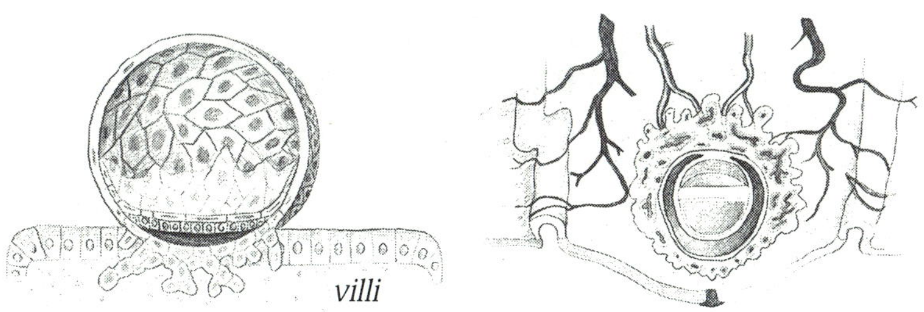

Second week *lining of womb*

Egg divides again and again to form blastocyst, which travels down Fallopian tube and implants in wall of the womb.

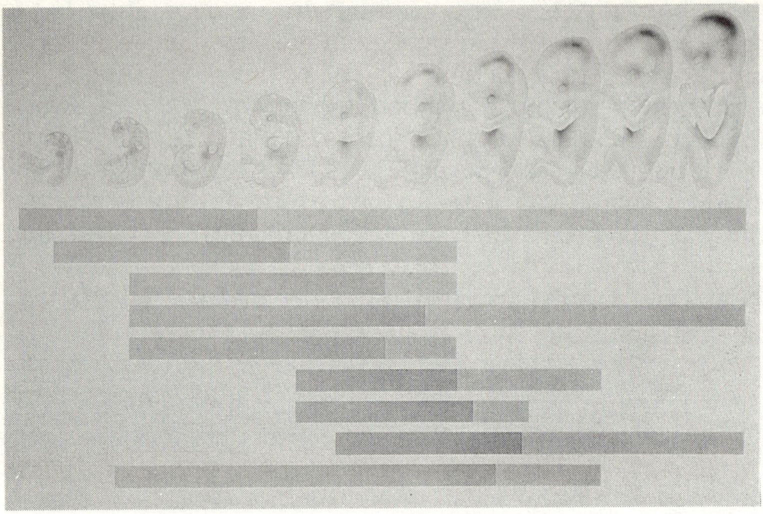

The light shading indicates when a particular organ starts to develop; the darker shading shows the most crucial stage in that development. (By permission Mother and Baby)

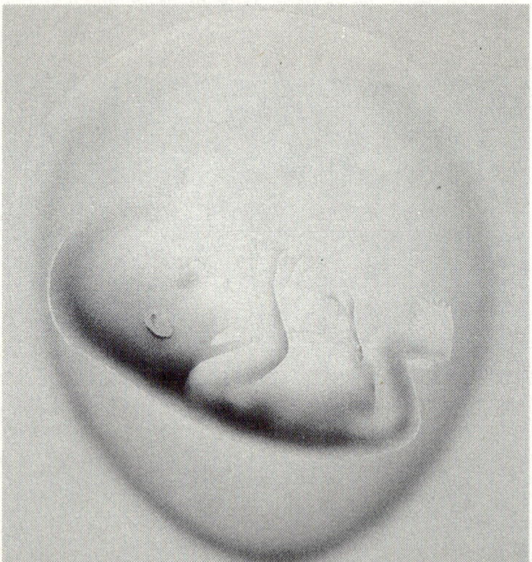

Long before you feel it, your baby is beginning to move: in the sixth week of life he moves his tiny arms and legs, and by the fourth month he can do nearly everything that a newborn baby can do. (Albert Lohr)

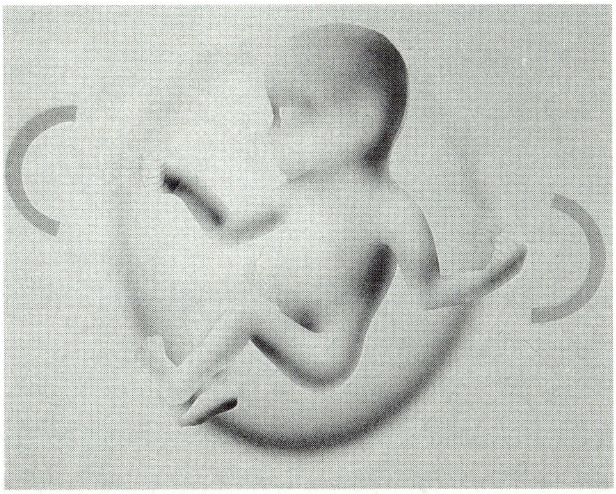

Towards the end of the fifth month, the unborn baby is about 25 cm long and weighs one pound. He's now so strong that you can easily feel his kicks and prods! He can hear now, too, and will react with strong kicking to loud noises such as cars hooting or rock music. (Albert Lohr)

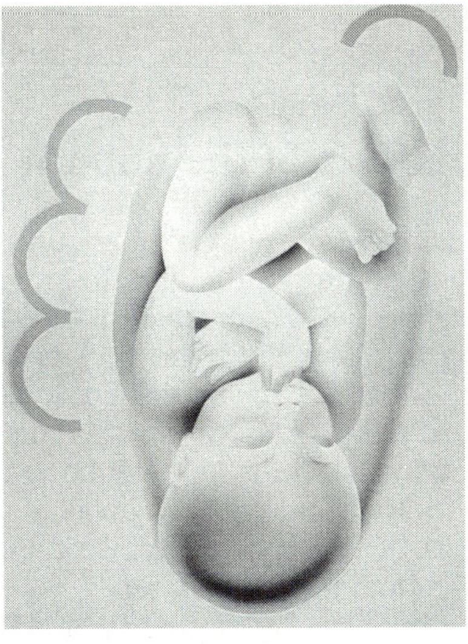

The nearer the birth approaches, the quieter the baby becomes. There's no room for somersaults any more. But when he stretches his legs a bit, it's easy to see the bulges on your abdominal wall. (Albert Lohr)

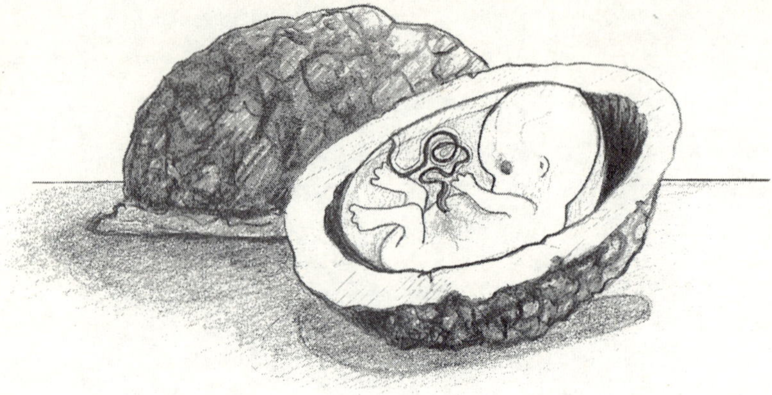

The human being at eight weeks would fit neatly into a walnut shell. Professor Jerome Lejeune, who is famous for his discovery of the extra chromosome in Down's Syndrome, suggests that the story of Tom Thumb was born out of a deep unconscious memory of the unborn baby at this size — i.e. less than a thumb's length from head to rump. Tom Thumb is one of those stories of little people (fairies, sprites, genii in bottles) that have universal appeal. The same stories turn up in many different countries and go back to antiquity. The fascination these stories exercise on us suggests that they reactivate feelings from the earliest and deepest parts of our psyches.

The needs of the unborn child

Technological equipment, such as ultrasound, has provided us with a fascinating picture of the growth and behaviour of the unborn child. We have also been able to study the growth of the premature baby from between the fifth and ninth month of gestation, when most normal babies are still in the womb.

The premature baby gives us an outside look at what is normally hidden inside. He is 'unplugged' from the biological rhythms of the mother and whisked away to an intensive care unit where he is deprived of the close contact which is so important for his healthy development.

Through a study of the premature baby we can get a pretty good idea of what is needed for the psychological and physical well-being of the unborn child from the fifth month until his birth. We can see what happens when mother and child are separated and the bonding process is interrupted. They are both put under tremendous stress; and the mother may feel that the child is no longer her own.

The sense of touch

We know what an unborn child feels, hears, sees, smells and tastes, and we know how his sense of touch develops. Of all the senses, the sense of touch is the most important and is the first to develop. You can survive without seeing or hearing, but not without a sense of touch. All other senses, in fact, could be said to be an extension of the sense of touch – seeing and hearing are 'touching' something at a distance from yourself, a kind of radar system allowing you to feel the presence of something with which you are not in direct physical contact. 'Touching' is also another word for loving. Often when we touch someone we are demonstrating our love for them. Our language recognizes this when we talk of being 'touched' by something – e.g. by words or actions.

I shall be explaining in a later chapter how you can feel and touch your unborn child, which is an expression of your love and care reinforces the bonding process.

The unborn child is responsive to pressure and touch. As early as nine weeks after conception, the fingers have developed well enough to wrap the palm of the hands round objects. At twelve weeks the child is able to close his fingers and thumb. He touches parts of his body with his hands and feet: early in pregnancy, when he accidentally touches an object he moves away from it; later he moves towards it.

He at first turns away from his hand when it touches his mouth, though the mouth opens. Later he opens his mouth and puts a finger or thumb in it. This is the rooting reflex which persists after birth: then it's usually the mother's nipple that touches the baby.

By the second month of gestation the baby will kick and jerk if poked at. If a needle touches him when a doctor is drawing off amniotic fluid to examine it for any signs of abnormality (during amniocentesis) the baby will jump and his heart rate will accelerate. In fact, the unborn child will react in the same way as a baby after birth to any kind of contact. He is highly sensitive to touch.

Hearing

It was once thought that the foetus was deaf and dumb. That was the state of our medical knowledge of prenatal life in the 19th century. We didn't know very much then; however, modern technology has opened our eyes to many things. As I have said, it has made us aware that the foetus is not the mindless creature once described in medical textbooks. Perhaps we should retain the medical term 'foetus' in a historical sense only for the description of what was once believed to be the condition of the unborn child: i.e. feeling nothing, hearing nothing and seeing nothing. The word 'foetus' does sound a bit like another useless bit of the body like an appendix. But how wrong we were about this tiny human being in the womb! How thoughtless we were! Now some people have such confidence in the unborn child's hearing ability that they sing and talk to him – and he actually responds! As a matter of fact, the unborn child has a completely developed auditory structure about half-way through pregnancy; and at birth a child's hearing is very acute and at least as good as an adult's. In the womb the baby responds to a wide range of sounds, some of them in frequencies so high or low that they cannot be heard by the adult ear. It has been suggested, however, that, because of this hyper-sensitivity, sensory pathways other than the ear may be involved.

Music

The unborn baby, who can hear many of the sounds that come to him from outside the womb, can, it seems, discriminate between various kinds of music, according to its rhythm or tempo. Michele Clements, a researcher at a London maternity hospital, found that the unborn child, at about four to five months, was soothed by Vivaldi and Mozart, but was disturbed by Beethoven, Brahms and rock. A baby, she said, will show his dislike of certain kinds of music by kicking wildly. But she may have been wrong about this. Perhaps the baby in the research failed to react to Vivaldi because of the absence of any strong beat, but was stimulated by rock. Although kicking is associated with anxiety, foetal movement is necessary for growth and it has been found that the unborn child sometimes moves in rhythm to music.

At any rate, Albert Liley found that from at least 25 weeks the unborn child would jump in rhythm with the timpanist's contribution to an orchestral performance. It may not, therefore, be so absurd, as it may sound to some, that a Liverpool doctor said that when his wife was pregnant he used to play the bagpipes a lot and that his unborn baby could be felt jumping or, as the doctor put it, 'dancing' to the sound of the music. Then when the boy was three or four years old he wanted to play the bagpipes. This may, of course, have been the result of the father's influence after birth, but the 'dancing' was probably a genuine response to the rhythm of the bagpipes.

It has been found that the newborn child likes sounds or music that mimic the whooshing sound he hears in the womb, which is how the beat of the heart comes to him. It's a soft sound like waves splashing on the beach, but with a distinctive rhythm. This is a sound that remains with us as a trace memory and has a fascination for us even as adults.

The Canadian Dr Thomas Verny recalls in his book, *The Secret Life of the Unborn Child* (Dell, New York, 1986), how he heard Boris Brott, conductor of the Hamilton (Ontario) Philharmonic Symphony, describe in an interview on the radio how he became interested in music. He said that as a young man he was mystified by the unusual ability he had to play certain pieces sight unseen. 'I'd be conducting a score for the first time,' he said, 'and suddenly the cello line would jump out at me; I'd know the flow of the piece before I found the page on the score. One day I mentioned this to my mother, who is a professional cellist. I thought she'd be intrigued because it was always the cello line that was so distinct in my mind. She was; but when she heard what the pieces were, the mystery quickly solved itself. All the scores I knew by sight were ones she had played while she was pregnant with me.'

The effect of music on the unborn child has been demonstrated by an Irish medical researcher, Dr Peter Hepper, who, in a letter to the British medical publication *The Lancet,* described a newborn baby's interest in a certain kind of TV music as Foetal Soap Addiction. Dr Hepper claims that babies of women who regularly watch TV soap operas during pregnancy respond immediately to the first bar of the soap opera's theme tune by focusing their rapt attention on the TV screen as the source of the sound.

There is no doubt that sound plays an important part in the life of the unborn child. This includes the sound of the human voice, especially the mother's voice, which the child recognizes immediately after birth. Singing lullabies to the unborn child is recommended by the British violinist Yehudi Menuhin, who believes that his own musical talent was partly due to the fact that his parents were always singing and playing music before he was born. Classes are now being held in prenatal bonding at various centres in the USA, including the Children's Hospital, Minnesota, which teach the mother to sing to her unborn child. I shall be discussing the role of sound in prenatal bonding, and suggesting how a mother can stimulate her unborn child by singing and talking to him, in a later chapter.

Vision

It has been discovered that, in spite of what doctors have been saying for years, a child's vision is well advanced at birth. It is quite remarkable that doctors have been so wrong about this. Even as late as 1964 a paediatric textbook (i.e. for child specialists) stated that newborn vision included little more than light sensitivity.

It is now known that a newborn's range of vision is about a foot or so. A change of light will change the size of the pupil. Pupils become constricted in the light and dilated in the darkness. Even in the dark the newborn will often scan the field and search for 'something to see' and his attention will finally move to particular targets. He can follow moving objects. His colour sense is very good and is essentially the same as that of an adult. He can discriminate between hues. He is intrigued with patterned surfaces, paying more attention to them than to plain surfaces. The newborn can also match sight with sound. His eyes will move towards the source of a sound that interests him as they did in the case quoted above of the baby with Foetal Soap Addiction.

All this indicates that visual ability is well developed in the womb. Muscles within the orbit are present very early in pregnancy and the eyes of the unborn child move during sleep and when he changes position. When a flash is used to photograph the abdomen, the unborn child is startled.

Any damage to the central nervous system during early

pregnancy could, among other things, affect the development of the eyes, so this is another reason why it is important for a mother to pay special attention to her health before conception and to avoid toxic substances that are known to cause neurological damage such as alcohol and nicotine.

Drinking

Amniotic fluid contains various chemicals including glucose, fructose, amino acids and salts. The unborn child drinks this fluid, which has a slightly chemical taste. On an average he drinks at the rate of 15 to 40 ml per hour in the last three months of pregnancy. There are, however, some who drink as much as 90 ml an hour. Large, well-nourished babies tend to drink at a high rate whereas small, skinny babies drink very little. The unborn child has a keen sense of taste. There are, in fact, more taste buds in his mouth than there are in the mouth of an infant or adult.

Albert Liley describes how the baby's drinking rate decreases dramatically following an injection of a solution called Lipidol 'K', which is a foul-tasting, iodinated poppy-seed oil which any adult or child would spit out in disgust. The unborn baby shows his dislike of any bitter taste by the sort of grimacing you might see on anyone's face who had just swallowed a spoonful of foul-tasting medicine. On the other hand, if a sweet taste such as saccharin is introduced into the amniotic fluid, he gulps it down with great relish. There are a few, however, who do not like the saccharin and probably find it bitter, as many adults do, when it is too concentrated.

Feeding habits before birth become the pattern after birth. A tardy drinker will be difficult to feed after birth; whereas a good drinker in the womb will also be a good drinker after birth. So the quality of the amniotic fluid is very important. The skinny baby in the womb, who is not well-nourished, will be difficult to feed after birth. Mothers who smoke, for instance, are in danger of producing small, skinny babies and this is likely to affect their drinking performance after birth: they will continue to be undernourished and susceptible to infections of various kinds.

Many women notice that their unborn baby sometimes has hiccups. This occurs at regular times and is associated with their baby's drinking. There are mothers who may be alarmed at this, particularly if there is a history of epilepsy in the family. They may mistake the hiccups for convulsions. But hiccups are very common and perfectly natural.

Sleeping and dreaming

The unborn baby, particularly during the last three months of pregnancy, has the same sleep patterns as the mother. This was demonstrated in some research carried out by the Swiss paediatrician, Stirnimann, who compared the sleep patterns of newborns of housewives with those of mothers with quite a different sleep cycle, who worked at night in bakeries. In each case the unborn baby had the same sleep pattern as the mother. A mother who changes her sleep pattern after birth will upset her baby and a mother who, during the last stage of pregnancy, keeps on getting up, or tossing and turning in bed during the night, may find after birth that the baby is disturbed at night and will keep parents awake.

There is evidence that we learn to dream in the womb. Electroencephalograph (EEG) examinations have shown that during sleep the unborn baby has rapid eye movements (REM), which in adults means that they are dreaming. The Austrian Dr Sepp Schindler is one of those who believe that the unborn child is in a dream-like state during these phases. His explanation for neurological activity during sleep – 'active sleep' – is that increasing restriction of movement experienced by the unborn child, as he grows during the last three months of pregnancy, is replaced by increasing activity in the brain. It may be a form of 'action replay', a visualization or rehearsal of movements learned in the womb that will be needed after birth. This, of course, is pure speculation. There are others who believe that dreaming is a mental exercise needed to facilitate the development of the central nervous system and its completion after birth. If this is so, it is important for a baby to get enough sleep, both before and after birth.

Premature babies spend more time dreaming than full term newborns. There are more smiles on the face of the premature baby than the full term newborn during REM/dream phases of sleep. REM/dreaming decreases as we grow older which seems to indicate that it is a mental activity related to physical activity. The less active we are, it seems, the less need we have for dreaming in adult life. However, this seems to contradict Dr Schindler's observation that the unborn child dreams during a period of diminished physical activity. Dreaming is generally thought to be concerned with a person's emotional life; and the more active an adult is, the more likely he is to be involved with others and to feel emotional stress at times. Vivid dreams occur at times of crisis, or when one feels repressed or denied an outlet for the expression of feelings. This would fit Schindler's theory of the unborn child feeling inhibited through restriction of movement. A biologist has described dreaming as the replaying of the DNA code, putting one back on course after a day's activity. No matter what it means, REM/dreaming seems to be important to the unborn child in the later stage of pregnancy.

Crying

A mother will understandably feel alarmed if she hears her baby crying in the womb, which sometimes happens. The cry occurs when air is brought into contact with the baby's larynx. The cry doesn't mean more than that. It is a sound, like the twanging of a guitar string, caused in the womb by an unusual occurrence. It used to happen in the days of air amniograms (to examine the inside of the womb) when, to prevent the crying, the mother was advised to stand in an upright position after examination.

Smell

Helen Keller described the sense of smell as 'a fallen angel'. Human beings have to a large extent lost the keen sense of smell that many animals have. The child, however, is still acutely sensitive to smell: to the scents that fill the air around him, the smell of food and the smell of his mother's skin, his father's clothes, the smell of every single thing: of tar bubbling between paving stones on a hot summer's day, the sweet smell of honeysuckle, the smell of lilac, roses, trees, the smell of the earth, the smell of towels, chairs, tables, toys. He is attracted or repelled by smell.

Smell is important in identifying what is good for you and what is poisonous. The smell of food cooking gets the gastric juices flowing. Newborns are particularly choosy about smells:

they are attracted to the odours of vanilla, strawberry, and banana (the sweet things in food that provide energy) and reject smells like ammonia and rotten fish. This olfactory sense develops in the womb. Soon after birth the baby will recognize the smell of his mother's breast pads, distinguishing them from plain or used pads of other mothers. The smell of the mother is very powerful. If the mother's diet is wholesome during pregnancy, and the chemistry of the womb is unadulterated, it will most certainly benefit the unborn child and may well have an effect on the child's subsequent eating habits.

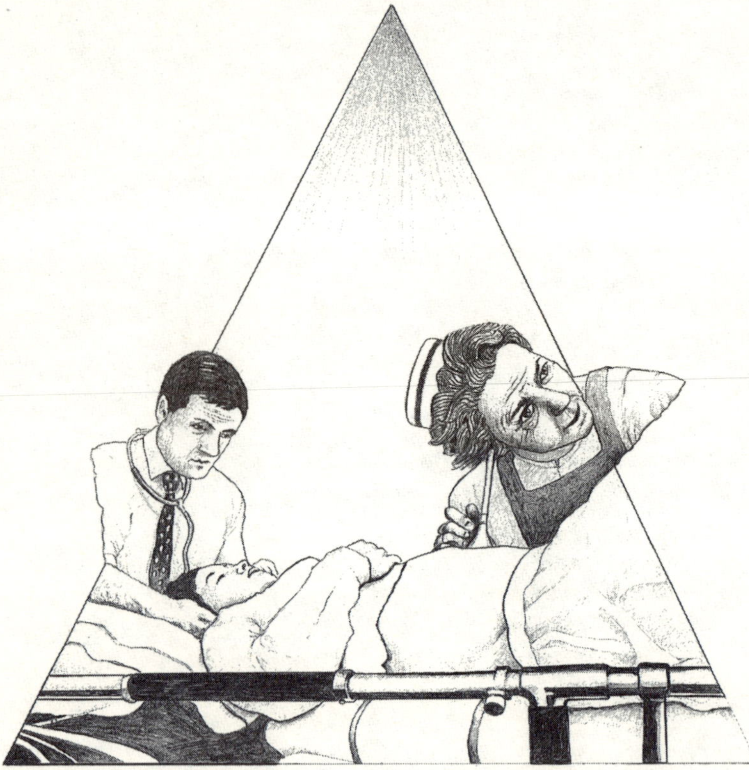

4

The baby at risk

How do I know my baby is all right, that nothing is going wrong in the way he is developing in the womb? How can I tell if there was any damage before I knew I was pregnant? What sort of illnesses can be inherited? Can epilepsy be inherited? If I've been smoking and drinking for years, is that going to harm my child? Is it all right to take aspirins? Will thrush harm the child? Or a heavy cold, or flu, or cystitis . . .? And what about depression? I feel anxious about my condition a lot of the time and my husband doesn't help . . . will that have a bad effect on my baby?

These are questions a mother might ask. For the majority of pregnancies it is unlikely that anything of a serious nature will or can go wrong. But the very fact that a mother asks questions about the possibility of bearing a handicapped child means that there is some nagging fear at the back of her mind. It is well to know what can go wrong and whether in her case there is any risk of a miscarriage, or whether her lifestyle or a history of some illness or disorder, such as epilepsy or diabetes, in her or her partner's family might put her child at risk. Any responsible prospective parent will consider this possibility, and will want to minimize any risk to the mother or child.

In the United Kingdom, in particular, the figures for infant mortality are high compared to many other Western countries. Even though most babies are born healthy, the risk of something going wrong is still higher than it should be. It is, in fact, estimated that one in seven pregnancies in Britain goes wrong. In 1988 over 6000 babies died before reaching their first birthday. In addition, there were 3549 miscarriages, and 47,848 low birth weight babies. Many of the deaths occurred in areas where there was high unemployment and substandard housing.

A study carried out by the British Office of Population Censuses and Surveys in 1988 showed how ill-health among people on low income was mainly due to their poor diet, plus factors such as smoking and drinking. However, the study also showed that other lifestyles produced other problems. For example, it was shown that breast, ovary and testicular cancer were more common in the higher income brackets. Women with higher incomes tended to have babies at a later age and this made them more vulnerable to breast cancer.

Whatever kind of lifestyle or income you have, the baby could be at risk if the parents lead a stressful life, especially if the mother, for economic reasons, has to continue to do work she doesn't like while she is pregnant, which so often happens these days. It is not a reason for giving up work, but it may be sensible to try to change your occupation, if you have any choice in the matter. The argument that a mother should stay at home for the sake of her child is a specious one. The home environment is not necessarily healthier than the work environment. In fact the pregnant woman might feel more depressed and sick at home than at work.

The effect of stress on the unborn child

Most pregnant women undergo shifts of mood and may be anxious at times. This is perfectly normal, and one must guard against adding to the pregnant woman's anxiety by overemphasizing the part stress plays in birth defects or complications during labour. There are techniques to reduce anxiety, which are discussed on page 68, but the best way of ensuring the health of the child is for both partners to adopt a healthy lifestyle, preferably before pregnancy.

Among the main causes of stress are: financial problems, being dissatisfied with your job, problems with relatives or previous relationships, a death in the family, the illness of a spouse, problems with friends, and religious differences, all or any of which may lead to marital difficulties. There is also the anxiety caused by an unwanted pregnancy, fear of responsibility or the fear of giving birth to a sick or handicapped child.

In most books about pregnancy the emphasis is usually put on the physical aspects, mainly as they affect the mother. While these are, of course, very important, you cannot separate them from psycho-social factors such as who the parents are, where they work, what their background is, and what their expectations are. All these things have a bearing on the health of parents and of the child.

We know a certain amount about the physical effect of acute emotional anxiety on the unborn child. We can, for example, through the help of ultrasound, observe his behaviour in the womb when the mother is emotionally disturbed. The highly anxious mother produces hyperactivity in the child, but we cannot say for certain what effect this might have on the child after birth. Common sense, however, tells us that it can't do him any good.

A mother sometimes knows intuitively if any harm is going to come to her child. It has been reported, for instance, that some mothers have known when they were going to have a miscarriage. There are those who claim that they are in touch, on a deep level, with the child and have dreams about losing him or can sense his predicament.

There are three main channels of communication with the unborn child: physiological, behavioural and what has been called 'sympathetic'. It is the 'sympathetic' that is least understood, mainly because it is difficult to measure in any conventional way.

Intuition plays a big part, as most mothers will testify, in the mother-child relationship. A good example of this is the way mothers in certain African tribes can sense when their babies need to urinate or defecate. The babies never wear nappies but never soil themselves. The mothers know exactly when to lift them off their hips and hold them over the road at the necessary times, without any obvious external signs. This sensitivity to the needs of a child is often lost to a mother who is suffering from emotional stress. It's true of any real problem. Unreal or psychological problems get in the way of the real problem. In fact, the inability to communicate with the unborn child — even if it's just a matter of visualization — and stress or anxiety go hand in hand. But I should not say *even* visualization: it has been found that the unborn child will sometimes respond in a physical way to a mother's image of him.

The unwanted pregnancy also causes stress and can be harmful to the unborn child. A study in Prague of 220 children born to mothers who had been refused abortions showed that there were serious differences in their psycho-social development, compared with an equal number of children who had been wanted. The children of the unwanted pregnancies grew up with feelings of deprivation or inadequacy. The study was followed through to adolescence and beyond, and it was found that feelings of inadequacy were passed on to the next generation.

Stress in itself is not necessarily injurious. It depends on how it is handled. To some people stress means stimulation. It's mainly when stress is intense and protracted and is accompanied by physical symptoms, such as reduced energy levels or insomnia, that it can be harmful, and lead to difficulties in pregnancy and a poor outcome.

Miscarriage

It is often said that a miscarriage occurs when the foetus is incapable of further development. Or, in other words, it is nature's way of terminating a pregnancy for the sake of the mother and child. Most women who have had miscarriages do not, as is commonly believed, necessarily have a defective reproductive system. The problem usually lies with the arrangement of chromosomes in the foetus, or in the ovum or sperm. Some research into the causes of miscarriages showed, in about 60 per cent of first-time pregnancies, that there was evidence of chromosomal disorders.

There is evidence that many miscarriages are caused by a poor diet, low in vitamins and minerals. This explains the link between poverty and miscarriage. Women on low incomes suffer more miscarriages than other women. Miscarriage that is not caused by some genetic or reproductive disorder is best prevented by living a healthy lifestyle. This means eating a well balanced diet which contains plenty of vitamins and minerals, with lots of vegetables and fruit, and avoiding alcohol and nicotine and non-prescribed medical drugs, some of which have been known to trigger off a miscarriage. And, most important, both parents should adopt a very positive attitude to the pregnancy and show as much interest in the unborn child as they do in their own health and peace of mind.

Genetic disorders

In most families there is some history of a particular type of illness. It may be a history of heart disease, cancer, neurological disorders, lung or stomach complaints. Some of these may be genetic; others may be caused by a particular kind of lifestyle that is handed down from one generation to the next. This is the concern of epidemiologists, who study the effect of the environment, lifestyle, or a culture, with its characteristic eating habits, on the incidence of a particular disease.

But there are genetic messages or flaws that may be handed down no matter who you are, or whether or not you live a healthy lifestyle. The most common of these include haemophilia and cystic fibrosis. There are others that are borderline — they may be inherited, but may arise spontaneously — such as diabetes or heart disease or some mental illness such as schizophrenia.

Haemophilia

This is a term applied to a group of blood disorders in which there is a life-long defect in the clotting factor which is known as factor VIII. In most cases there is a family history of the disease, but there are a few cases where the haemophiliac is first in the line. The most common disorder is classical haemophilia, which is transmitted by both sexes but causes bleeding only in the male, except in rare circumstances. In the past 10-15 years effective treatment has been available for haemophiliacs and sufferers can now lead relatively normal lives and expect to marry and have children of their own.

Prenatal diagnosis is now available. A blood sample can be taken from a male foetus, at 18-20 weeks of pregnancy, by means of foetoscopy, to determine if the boy has haemophilia. If there is a risk of haemophilia, it is best for the parents to decide before pregnancy whether they are prepared to take that risk, and if the test proves positive, are they prepared to make the agonizing decision of aborting the child?

Muscular dystrophy

Another sex-linked genetic disease is a form of muscular

dystrophy known as the Duchenne type. This type affects only boys, although other types of muscular dystrophy affect both sexes. Boys who are born with Duchenne's disease lose their ability to walk between the ages of four and ten, and are usually confined to wheelchairs during their short lives.

Cystic fibrosis (CF)

This is a genetic condition which affects one in every 2000 babies in the Western world. One in twenty Caucasians (white Europeans as well as those from India and the Middle East) is a carrier of the CF gene, and when this is present in both parents there is a one in four chance that any child of theirs will inherit the disease. The CF gene was identified in July, 1989. This was the end of ten years' painstaking, intensive research, but also the start of new research which, it is expected, will result in truly effective treatment for every person born with CF. Pharmacologists are trying to design drugs to alter the fault in the membrane transport which has been revealed by the faulty gene. It is estimated that it will be another five to ten years before an effective drug is developed. Carrier testing is now available. This takes the form of either blood spot or mouth wash analysis, which is quicker and more accurate than previous testing. Prenatal diagnosis can also be carried out, and if tests prove positive abortion is offered at eleven weeks of gestation.

The disease mainly affects the lung and digestive system. The main characteristic is the thick and sticky mucus, which accumulates in the lungs and must be cleared by regular physiotherapy (postural drainage). CF patients also have to take antibiotics regularly to reduce the germs that tend to multiply in the lung secretions. The mucus also blocks the ducts of various organs, in particular the pancreas, where it blocks the flow of digestive enzymes and, if not treated, results in malnutrition. The enzymes are replaced by pancreatic secretions from an animal which are taken in the form of tablets or powder before meals. The condition can be very distressing both for the parents and child, depending on its severity, which varies widely. The treatment, however, has greatly improved since CF was first diagnosed in 1938, and now many patients reach adulthood and some of them marry and have children of their own, who are not affected by the disease if the partner is not a carrier. Men with CF however, are very often sterile, due to a blockage of the duct that carries the seminal fluid.

Down's Syndrome

This is a chromosomal disorder, caused when an egg cell (or sometimes a sperm cell) has a certain chromosome (known as number 21) in duplicate, so that the fertilized egg has 47 instead of the usual 46 chromosomes. Down's Syndrome affects one in every 1000 births. The Down's Syndrome baby has the typical facial characteristics of slanting eyes (which is why the condition was once called mongolism), small features and a large tongue that often sticks out. The back of the head is usually flat.

The baby is usually mentally handicapped, and has to go to a special school. But many parents of Down's Syndrome children say what a joy they are, and how pleased they are that they didn't decide on having an abortion. These children are responsive, loving and even-tempered, and many are fond of music. A blood test is now available early in pregnancy which will show if there is a possibility that your baby has Down's Syndrome. It still has to be confirmed later in pregnancy — in the test known as amniocentesis. But for those who are not affected, the fear is removed early in pregnancy. It is the older woman who will ask for the test, because the risk of having a baby with this abnormality increases in women over the age of 35.

Familial hypercholesterolaemia (FH)

This is the medical term for an inherited condition in which the blood cholesterol levels are so high that there is a risk of heart attacks and other complications caused by the hardening of the arteries. The condition affects one in 500 people. If one parent has the FH gene, the chances are that half the children will inherit it. Such individuals are known as heterozygotes. FH can be detected at birth by a test in which a sample of umbilical cord blood is taken. The condition is treated with a diet of low cholesterol, low saturated fat (found in dairy products) and high polyunsaturated fat. Such people should never smoke nor take contraceptive pills without medical advice.

Polygenic disorders

These are a group of disorders caused by a genetic flaw

combined with environmental factors. Some seem to be triggered by viruses, vitamin and mineral deficiencies or even by the seasons of the year. In the Northern hemisphere polygenic disorders are more common in babies conceived in the spring and born in the winter. The most common disorders in this group include cleft lip and/or palate, congenital dislocation of the hip, pyloric stenosis (a narrowing of the intestine where it leaves the stomach), or what is commonly called hole in the heart. All of these disorders can be remedied by surgery.

Two of the most serious of polygenic disorders are *spina bifida* and *hydrocephalus.* They are disorders of the central nervous system, which is one of the first parts of the body to develop when the embryo is 20 days old and a groove appears in the centre of what will be the baby's back. This groove deepens and the edges above it join to form a tube known as the neural tube. The front part expands to form the brain; the back part becomes the spinal cord.

Spina bifida and hydrocephalus are known as neural tube defects because they are caused by something that goes wrong in the early development of the central nervous system when the tube is forming.

Spina bifida is a defect in part of the bony spine that helps to protect the spinal cord. The nerves in that area — usually the lower spine — are exposed and unprotected and may also be defective. These nerves control the muscles of the legs, bladder and bowels and a child with the defect may have some paralysis of the legs and incontinence. There are, however, others who are only mildly affected and may have hardly any physical handicap.

Hydrocephalus (also known as water on the brain) is a swelling of internal brain spaces (ventricles) which makes the head grow larger than normal. The defect can be detected in the womb by means of X-ray or ultrasound. If the defect is well advanced before birth, it may be necessary, for the mother's own safety, to deliver the child by Caesarean section. If the defect is not too advanced, it can be relieved after birth by an operation.

It has been found that in families where one child has spina bifida, a recurrence is prevented in a second pregnancy by the administration of multi-vitamin tablets, folic acid, iron and minerals. One study in South Wales suggested that folic acid alone may help to reduce the risk of recurrence.

It is thought probable that a deficiency in some essential nutrients in the pregnant woman's diet, and/or, in some cases, toxification by nicotine, alcohol and other environmental poisons contributes to the occurrence of polygenic disorders.

Ethnic Disorders

Different ethnic groups are susceptible to certain kinds of genetic disorders. For example, the most common form of genetic disease in blacks is sickle cell anaemia, so-called because of the sickle-shaped red blood cells it produces, which contain defective haemoglobin, an essential iron-carrying protein. The disease, which affects one in 400 blacks, causes the clogging of small blood vessels and may result in a stroke. Those with the disease are also susceptible to meningitis and other serious infections, and chronic illness may be expected. But, as with cystic fibrosis, patients can, with care, live a productive life despite ill-health.

One or both of two types of thalassaemia (alpha and beta) are common among blacks, Asians and people of Mediterranean stock. This also produces anaemia and chronic ill-health. Blood transfusions may be necessary. Not all cases are severe; some patients may survive for many years.

Ty-Sachs disease is a genetic disorder which sometimes occurs among Ashkenazic Jews. It is a fatal condition resulting in the deterioration of the brain. Few children with the disease live beyond five years. No adequate treatment is known.

Genetic counselling

If you have any fear that a family illness or genetic disorder could be passed on to your unborn child, you should consult a genetic counsellor. Your family doctor or obstetrician will be able to refer you to your nearest genetics centre.

Illnesses, apart from genetic diseases, and various infections that may put your child at risk are described on page 66.

Tests for genetic disorders

In recent years there has been an explosion of high-tech procedures which are carried out to test if the unborn baby has any abnormalities or illness. The tests are not a hundred per cent safe, but for pregnant women who are at risk and for the unborn child who is sick there are undoubted benefits. Our knowledge of the life of the unborn baby has improved considerably as a result of ultrasound. But the indiscriminate use of high-tech procedures may create problems that are worse than the ones they were designed to solve.

Ultrasound

This is the commonest test which enables the doctor – and you – to look at your unborn child. An image appears on a TV screen as the result of bouncing sound waves off the baby.

Ultrasound was welcomed as an alternative to X-rays for investigating various medical conditions – eg. abnormalities of early pregnancy – the gestational age of the unborn baby, or to confirm multiple pregnancies. It was considered a fairly safe procedure compared with X-rays. Nowadays, however, ultrasound for many doctors has become a routine procedure. For the parents, seeing the child in the womb helps them to relate to him and is reassuring to parents who have fears about whether their unborn child is normal or not, as some do, even though the baby or mother is not considered to be at risk.

There are, however, warnings by medical researchers that ultrasound could cause genetic damage, though there is no conclusive proof of this. In 1984 the USA National Institutes of Health issued a report which discouraged the use of ultrasound 'solely to satisfy the family's desire to know the foetal sex, to view the foetus, or to obtain a picture of the foetus.'

Amniocentesis

This is a test carried out between 16 and 20 weeks to establish if your baby has any chromosomal disorder. Analysis of foetal cells found in the amniotic fluid around the baby will reveal, for instance, whether the child has Down's Syndrome, which is the reason why an older woman usually has the test. It is also used to diagnose neural tube defects such as spina bifida. In most cases the test proves negative.

The fluid is taken out with a needle inserted in the abdominal wall under local anaesthetic. Ultrasound is used to make sure the needle is inserted in the right place and does not harm the baby or placenta. Although the risk of complications is slight, they can be serious, and may even result in the death of the baby. Furthermore, amniocentesis is not always satisfactory: the sample of amniotic fluid may be unreliable or the laboratory analysis may be wrong.

The whole object of the test is to give parents the opportunity to terminate a pregnancy if some serious abnormality is discovered. But there are parents who would regard 16-20 weeks as too late to have an abortion, and they may be offered chorion villus sampling (CVS) at an earlier stage of pregnancy.

CVS

This test can be carried out in the tenth week of pregnancy. There is a slight risk of miscarriage, estimated at 1-4 per cent. A sample is taken from the chorion villus, which is a mass of cells surrounding the amniotic sac, and later develops into the placenta. The test takes about ten minutes from start to finish. It may be followed by a dull 'period' pain. The long wait for the results – sometimes as long as a fortnight – can be an anxious time. But if, as is likely, the result is negative, you may consider it all worthwhile. If it is positive, then making a decision about an abortion can be just as agonizing as it is later on. Whether the child is big or small, you are destroying a life. This has to be faced; and if, for any reason, you are considered at risk, it is better to face the possibility of having to abort your child before pregnancy rather than afterwards when a child is actually on the way. Both partners should be prepared for this.

Foetoscopy

In this test a needle containing a fine telescope is inserted through the abdomen into the womb, and the doctor can look through this at the baby or take a blood sample to test for disorders that cannot be detected through amniotic fluid cells. The procedure may also be used for medical treatment of the unborn child, including blood transfusions.

Foetoscopy is a riskier procedure than amniocentesis or chorion villus sampling, resulting in miscarriages in some 3-5 per cent of pregnancies. There are other risks, including leakage of amniotic fluid during the later months of pregnancy, infection and the scarring of the womb.

One benefit of the procedure is that it is making obstetricians more sensitive to the presence of the baby in the womb. One obstetrician was reported as saying: 'I had a blood vessel lined up and was just about to strike when out of nowhere came this hand to knock away the needle. I think it was coincidental, but who knows?'

Treating the unborn child

The unborn child can now be treated for a number of disorders and illnesses. Enzyme deficiencies in the unborn child and other abnormalities of metabolism, growth or development, can be treated through a diet that puts back the missing nutrients or hormones or prevents toxins from being absorbed.

Hydrocephalus has been treated by inserting a 'shunt' in the brain to relieve pressure caused by the build-up of cerebrospinal fluid. There is a success rate of about 25 per cent in these operations. Some conditions such as Rh incompatibility (see page 70) and heart rhythm irregularities can be detected and treated in the womb.

Metabolic illnesses and infections

There are a number of metabolic illnesses and infections that can put mother and baby at risk. The most serious of these are as follows.

Diabetes

Most women with diabetes can have children, but they need special care during pregnancy, and they should make every effort to keep their blood glucose level under control right from the time of conception to the time of delivery. In the past, about a third of the babies born to women with diabetes were lost. Now, with good care, the chances of losing a baby are only slightly greater than for those who do not have diabetes. There are, however, still a few women with long-standing diabetes, raised blood pressure, and kidney problems, who are generally advised against pregnancy because of the high risk of an unsatisfactory outcome.

Diabetes is one of those conditions where preconceptual care is advisable. If you are planning to start a family, or have another child, you should inform your doctor, or your diabetic clinic, just in case there should be any reason why pregnancy is, in your case, an unacceptable risk. You should aim at getting your diabetic control near-perfect before pregnancy. A diabetic father should do the same for the sake of his own health, but his control does not increase the risk of any abnormality in the child.

During pregnancy it will probably be necessary to visit your doctor or diabetic clinic every two to four weeks. Frequent tests are important and your insulin requirement is likely to increase during pregnancy. It is also very important to pay attention to your diet, and make sure that it includes all the necessary nutrients to help build a healthy baby and to keep up your own energy and resistance to infection.

Diabetes developing during pregnancy

Sometimes diabetes is discovered for the first time during a routine test which the pregnant woman undergoes. This is known as 'gestational diabetes' and in most cases the problem is resolved as soon as the baby is delivered. The treatment, however, is exactly the same as for long-standing diabetes, and it is important to maintain control of the blood glucose level throughout pregnancy. The likelihood is that diabetes will recur during subsequent pregnancies, so it is important that you should report this problem to your doctor the moment you think you are pregnant.

The Diabetic Handbook (Insulin Dependent) includes an up-to-date and comprehensive chapter on pregnancy. It is published by Thorsons and the British Diabetic Association (BDA). Copies can be obtained from the BDA (see address in the Resources section).

High Blood Pressure

Like diabetes, persistent high blood pressure is a condition that calls for special care before and during pregnancy. However, with many pregnant women who normally don't have a blood pressure problem, it is very difficult to get a true measurement because blood pressure can rise for a variety of emotional and environmental reasons. It can go shooting up sometimes at an antenatal clinic. If it's any consolation to those who suffer in this way, it is quite a common occurrence. For most women there's a slight rise of blood pressure during pregnancy anyway; and a visit to the antenatal clinic or the doctor, particularly in the early stages, are anxious moments, so any dramatic rise in blood pressure is likely to be only temporary. A study of 48 patients reported in *The Lancet* showed that in every case blood pressure rose sharply at the beginning of every visit to a doctor.

However, if you are worried that you may have a blood pressure problem, you should consider home recording. Your doctor will give you advice on taking your blood pressure at home. At the Rosie Maternity Hospital in Cambridge, out-patients who are considered to be at risk because of high blood pressure are taught to operate an automated blood pressure monitor. The blood pressure is transmitted to the hospital by telephone two or three times a day and displayed on a VDU screen. The obstetrician keeps a check on the patient's blood pressure and can decide when or if to admit a patient to hospital. But this is only in high risk cases.

Alternative medical practitioners offer various remedies for high blood pressure. Many pregnant women have found meditation very helpful. Acupuncture can also be used to treat high blood pressure. A herbal remedy for normalizing both high and low blood pressure is one teaspoon of Cayenne, three times a day in orange juice or yoghurt.

For everyone, whether at risk or not, relaxation exercises can help in the prevention or treatment of high blood pressure. Relaxation is mainly a matter of letting go. The problem is in the mind, but the solution is mainly in the body where muscles tense up. By focusing attention on what is going on in your body, you turn the mind away from its worries.

You begin by focusing attention on the feet. Wriggle your toes, bend your ankles upwards; tense every part of the feet and then let go. Feel the feet getting warm. Then move your attention up your legs to your calves. Tense the calves; then let go. Then move up to the knees, and so on all the way up the body. Feel the blood coursing through your veins. It is a good idea to do this to some appropriate quiet music that has the effect of filling you with delicious sensations of peace and love. In any case, during pregnancy you should fill your home with music. It's therapeutic on its own, good for you, your partner and your baby and certainly a good way of getting rid of tensions. Choose the sort of music you can flop into.

Relaxation training is important for both partners as a part of childbirth training. It makes you aware of your body, teaching you to recognize anxiety and fear in muscular tensions. It teaches you control over your body. The mere recognition of tension sometimes leads, through what is known as passive control, to its reduction without your doing anything consciously.

As in the treatment of other conditions, a good diet and nutrition and a healthy lifestyle with adequate rest and relaxation, and giving up smoking and alcohol, of course, are effective ways of preventing and treating high blood pressure. But if you have a problem, don't imagine you can get along entirely on your own without professional advice. Make sure your doctor is kept informed about what you are doing for it. He or she will probably approve of anything that helps you to relax, but will warn you if there's any sign of illness, which may need special treatment.

Pre-eclampsia

A sudden rise in blood pressure may indicate that you have pre-eclampsia (pre-eclampsia toxaemia or PET) which is a condition that affects between five and ten per cent of women in the last three months of pregnancy, and is fairly common in a first pregnancy. Besides high blood pressure, other symptoms are an excess of protein in the urine, swollen ankles and fingers due to water retention.

A test you can do for yourself is to press your skin firmly and if the mark it makes stays indented longer than usual, you may have pre-eclampsia. If you have any of these symptoms, you should consult a doctor or midwife immediately. A mild case can be cured quite easily with bed rest and it won't affect the unborn baby, but if it is neglected, it could develop into full-blown eclampsia, which sends the mother into convulsions and can be dangerous for her and her unborn baby. This, however, rarely happens if the first onset of symptoms are dealt with promptly.

A poor diet is believed by many experts to be an important factor in causing pre-eclampsia. They agree that a well-balanced diet each day from a wide variety of nourishing foods is the best protection against pre-eclampsia. The Pre-eclampsia Toxaemia (PET) Society, which is a self-help and support group for sufferers, favours the diet recommended by Dr Tom Brewer, the American specialist in maternal and child health, who believes that the pregnant woman should eat a high-protein diet with salt as desired and no restriction on weight gain providing you are eating the right kind of food.

Rubella or German measles

This common infection is a serious threat to the unborn child. Rubella in children or adults is a relatively harmless infection causing no more inconvenience than a common cold, but it can cause deformities in the unborn child during the first three months of pregnancy. To protect your child it is advisable to take precautions before pregnancy – i.e. before the use of contraceptives is discontinued. Get your rubella immunity checked. Even if you have been immunized in the past, the antibodies may not be at full strength, and you may need another injection.

Toxoplasmosis

A very infectious disease caused by the organism *Toxoplasma gondii*, which lives in the intestines of dogs and cats and is found in their faeces. It is present in some 20 to 30 per cent of all American women and even more Western Europeans. If the mother becomes infected during the first three months of pregnancy, the child can suffer serious abnormalities such as hydrocephalus (water on the brain) or brain malformation.

The best protection against the infection is to keep pets indoors as much as possible, feed them only prepared foods, and always wash animal and human eating utensils separately. Don't handle litter boxes and don't allow your pets to lick you. Raw meat may be a source of infection, so take care when preparing meat for cooking, and make sure it is thoroughly cooked before eating. Keep raw meat in separate containers in the fridge.

Rhesus (Rh) disease

This is a disease in which a mother with Rh negative cells in her blood will form antibodies to a baby's Rh positive cells inherited from the father. The baby will suffer from severe anaemia, jaundice, and possibly heart failure before it is born. Pregnant women are routinely tested to see if they are Rh negative. Fortunately Rh disease is now becoming rare because an anti-D immunoglobulin injection, which can be given within 27 hours of giving birth, prevents the formation of antibodies.

Sexually transmitted diseases

Gonorrhoea, syphilis and AIDS are the most serious of the sexually transmitted diseases. If either parent has cause to believe that he or she may be infected, a frank discussion before planning a family is absolutely necessary. If there are any doubts, a doctor should be consulted. It is rare for a woman to become pregnant when suffering from gonorrhoea because it causes acute inflammation of the Fallopian tubes, which causes considerable damage to the tissues and blockage of the tubes. If treated in its very early stage, before the tubes are damaged, it can be cured. A very small number of women do become pregnant when suffering from gonorrhoea, or they contract the disease during pregnancy. A child infected with gonorrhoea, often has serious eye infections and there is a risk of blindness.

Syphilis is more devastating. In pregnancy syphilis in its first two stages will lead to premature birth, stillbirth or death of the newborn. Fortunately antibiotics have made it extremely rare for syphilis to develop to the third (tertiary) stage which leads to a complete breakdown of body functions. At this stage it has devastating effects on all the organ systems of the unborn child.

A pregnant woman is given a blood test when she first visits the antenatal clinic and this will establish whether or not she is suffering from syphilis.

AIDS (or the Acquired Immune Deficiency Syndrome) is caused by a virus called immunodeficiency virus or HIV. Not everyone infected with the virus goes on to develop AIDS, which suggests that other factors are involved. Alcohol, high stress levels, and frequent exposure to other disease, particularly sexually transmitted diseases, have been suggested as possibilities.

No one should start a family if there is any fear of being HIV positive and passing on the infection to the child. A simple test will establish whether you are infected. It is important that, when preparing for pregnancy, couples should be completely honest with each other about previous sexual liaisons or drug abuse.

Herpes simplex infections

There are two types of herpes simplex virus: HSV 1, which appears as cold sores on the face, usually around the lips and mouth; and HSV 2, or herpes genitalis, which mainly affects the genital area and appears as small blisters which burst to leave small, red painful ulcers. Herpes genitalis affects both sexes and is caught during sexual intercourse with a person whose genitals are infected or after oral sex with someone who has cold sores.

Herpes simplex infections can never be cured: the virus hides in the tissues and remains there for the whole of the sufferer's life. It usually erupts when a person is run down as a result of stress, a poor diet, or consuming too much alcohol and other drugs. A woman who is subject to herpes simplex infections needs to look after herself extremely well during pregnancy. Swabs should be taken from the vagina in the last few weeks of pregnancy to ensure that the virus is not actively present. If it is, then a Caesarian section will be recommended because there is a 50 per cent chance that the baby will die if he or she contracts the disease during vaginal delivery.

Common minor problems of pregnancy

Morning sickness

Morning sickness is quite a puzzling condition. In the first place, it's not really an appropriate description because less than one tenth of women are sick in the early morning only. It can happen at any time of the day. And in the second place, no one knows for certain what brings it on; but whatever it is, the baby is doing it to you. The baby is asking you to take care. The sickness can vary in intensity, ranging from mild nausea to vomiting. It's called a 'minor' complaint but it can make you feel very ill and miserable. Because it's regarded as a 'minor' illness and has no harmful long-term effects on you or your baby, very little research has been carried out into its cause. One theory links morning sickness with high levels of a hormone known as HGC (human chorionic gonadotrophin) in the blood. The hormone passes out into the urine and its presence is what makes your pregnancy test positive.

Another theory is that it has a nutritional cause. Maybe the baby is not getting all the nutrients he needs or is getting too much of the wrong foods. The most severe forms of morning sickness occur in women whose diet is high in protein and low in carbohydrates.

Various treatments are recommended. As with any illness

which causes stress, accepting it and not feeling guilty about it or talking about it to a friend or relative can help. If you feel sick in the morning, you should start your day very slowly. A cup of tea and some dry toast or a cracker before getting up can help. You should start by nibbling the toast or cracker very slowly before you sit up. Sitting up suddenly can bring on the sickness. The nausea gets worse on an empty stomach so eating little and often may be preferable to large regular meals.

The Bircher-Benner approach (see page 151) is dietary, concentrating on raw and fresh food. They suggest that on waking you should eat a few raisins or pine kernels. It can also help to chew mint and peppermint leaves.

If the problem is a weakness in the stomach and digestive system and your tongue is white or pale and covered with mucus, a ginger drink (¼oz/6g of Root Ginger to a pint of water sweetened with honey) has been found helpful. You could also try an infusion of raspberry leaves.

If the cause of the problem is the liver, your pulse will feel 'wiry' and a yellowish tongue with red parts round the edges. In this case try infusions made from Gentian, Balm Melissa or a weak mint tea.

The problem usually disappears in the 13th or 14th week. But then it may be replaced by indigestion or heartburn.

Heartburn

This has nothing to do with the heart. It gets its name from the fiery sensations which seem to be near the heart and are caused by the action of the pregnancy hormone progesterone relaxing the valve at the upper end of the stomach which prevents the regurgitation of food and stomach acids. It is aggravated in late pregnancy by the pressure of the enlarging womb on the stomach and gullet.

It is important to avoid rich, greasy and spicy foods and alcohol (which can damage your baby) and you should resist the temptation of tucking into a large meal just before going to bed. Heartburn is exacerbated by bending or lying flat; it helps to sleep propped up on pillows.

It is not advisable to take large doses of a strong alkaline mixture, which only relieves the symptoms for a short time and tends to make things worse because the stomach reacts to alkali by producing increasing amounts of acid. A milk drink with slippery elm can help.

If the heartburn becomes severe and resistant to any of the above suggestions, you should see a doctor who will probably prescribe an effective antacid. But avoid medicines containing aluminium, which may harm the baby. Evidence is building up that aluminium is a neuro-toxin that may damage the central nervous system of the unborn child.

Constipation

This is very common in pregnancy and is also sometimes caused by the relaxing effect of progesterone – but this time on the smooth muscle of the intestine. The best treatment is a diet of fresh fruit and vegetables and high fibre foods, including wholemeal bread, which your baby is demanding. But go easy on the bran because it can prevent the absorption of iron. If all else fails, try lavish helpings of prunes, figs and grapes. Constipation combined with headaches may be caused by dehydration, so drink plenty of liquids.

Piles or haemorrhoids

These may be caused by constipation and straining. Piles, which are actually varicose veins in the back passage, usually start with irritation and itching. They can be quite painful. They usually disappear after your baby is born. In the meantime you can avoid them by preventing constipation, or if you do become constipated, you should treat it sensibly and avoid straining, which happens when you panic after a day or so.

There are various ointments (such as Anusol) for the relief of piles, which you can get from your chemist. A warm bath is also helpful.

Varicose veins

These are very painful, causing your legs to ache and throb. They occur when the veins of the legs become wide and slack and there is a breakdown of valves, which leads to swelling. As the pregnancy advances the pressure on the pelvic veins tends to block the flow of blood from the legs to the heart, thus increasing the pressure within the veins of the legs.

There are some doctors who will supply support tights on prescription. These should be put on immediately after getting up in the morning. Varicose veins can be prevented by gentle exercise, never standing still and never crossing your legs. Excessive weight gain doesn't do you any good, of course; but before you start cutting down on calories to reduce your weight, you should get professional advice. You should put your feet up as often as you can, keeping your heels above the level of your hips.

Thrush or Candida albicans

We all carry a parasitic yeast or fungus in our bodies, which usually doesn't bother us, but becomes active as a result of a poor diet, smoking, the consumption of alcohol and the over-use of antibiotics, which can damage your health and your baby's. It can also be aggravated by perfume, hairsprays or petrol fumes.

The symptoms include intense itching around the vagina and a white, curdy discharge. The treatment is to cut out yeast products, wine, mushrooms and cheese. Live yoghurt is particularly effective, so eat plenty of it and apply it to the affected part. Garlic is also recommended. You can take it in capsules called perles, which you should take three or four times a day. Alternatively, you can insert a peeled clove in the vagina at night. Thrush is essentially a disease of an impaired immune system, indicating that there is a need for cultivating a more healthy lifestyle. Dr Alfred Vogel, the Swiss nutritionist, recommends in his book *Viruses, Allergies and the Immune System* (Mainstream Publishing, 1988) that you take the following supplementary vitamins daily whenever the immune system is under threat:

- vitamin C (1–2 g)
- B-complex (yeast free)
- zinc (50–100 mg)
- magnesium (300–400 mg)
- vitamin E (200–400 IU)
- selenium (50 mg)
- folic acid (30 mg)
- vitamin A (10,000–15,000 IU).

Vaginal discharges

These sometimes get worse during pregnancy and although they can be a nuisance, this is quite normal. If the discharge is thick and itchy or has an unpleasant smell, you should consult your doctor. You probably have an infection. The two commonest are thrush, described above, or trichomonas, which is a greenish discharge and sometimes has a fishy smell. Trichomonas is usually treated by a course of antibiotics. Some of these infections thrive in the vaginal area because it is usually warm and airless, so always wear light cotton underwear, which is cooler and more absorbent than synthetic fibres. Avoid tights and nylon briefs.

Cystitis

This is a very common ailment, which is caused by bacteria travelling up from the urethra into the bladder. Though it can be distressing, it doesn't normally present a serious health risk. The main symptom is the frequent urge to urinate, but when you try to do so only a small amount of urine is passed. Urinating is painful and has been described as '. . . like passing broken glass'.

About 20 per cent of women have bacteria present in their urine, which some experts blame on a poor diet. The following dietary regime should help.

On the first day don't eat anything at all, but drink the following:

- Four pints (2 litres) of water with a teaspoon of sodium bicarbonate per pint (½ litre). The fluids flush away the germs and sodium bicarbonate makes the urine less acid and prevents bacteria from multiplying.
- Soup of strained liquid in which barley and vegetables have been cooked.

Note: if you are subject to high blood pressure, you should consult your doctor before taking bicarbonate of soda. Otherwise, maintain this diet until the symptoms subside. Then follow this diet by adding brown rice, vegetables and fish and gradually return to a normal diet, but avoid meat, which is acidic, until you are symptom-free.

If this fails, you should consult your doctor who may prescribe a course of antibiotics. Hygiene, of course, is important. As with thrush, the organisms that cause cystitis thrive in a warm and airless atmosphere, so wear loose-fitting clothes, preferably made of cotton.

Muscle cramps in the legs

These are quite common in pregnancy. The best treatment is to get out of bed and massage the affected muscles vigorously. Another treatment that is often recommended is to hold your toes and pull them up towards you. You could also try standing with your feet flat on the floor and leaning towards the wall. It is believed that cramps may be caused by calcium deficiency. You may not be eating enough foods rich in calcium, such as dairy products.

Backache

This is another very common condition during pregnancy, and again the culprit is usually the hormone progesterone which relaxes ligaments that support the spinal column. The problem is exacerbated by the strain your extra weight puts on the back. The best way to avoid this is by correcting your posture before pregnancy by exercises such as the Alexander Technique (see page 28). Sit straight up in a chair; don't slouch. Don't bend forwards to lift anything; try to keep your back straight as you kneel down. Ask your partner or a friend to massage your back gently. Wear low-heeled shoes and go barefoot indoors as much as possible. Sleep on a firm mattress. Adequate rest is also important, especially during the last three months of pregnancy.

Tiredness

There is often a complete sapping of energy during the first three weeks of pregnancy when 'three o'clock feels like nine o'clock at night'. The way to deal with this is not to fight it, but to take a nap whenever you can. If you are still at work, you should try to alter your hours so that you avoid the morning and evening rush hours which can be so exhausting at the best of times, but can completely knock you out during the early weeks and later stages of pregnancy. If you are used to a lot of entertaining and staying up late, you should realize that you can no longer do this and must give up the late nights and arrange for at least a few early nights a week. Some women are helped by oil of Evening Primrose capsules. The tiredness disappears in the middle months of pregnancy, but returns towards the end when the physical demands are great and you may have sleepless nights because you can't find a comfortable position in bed and are kept awake by the baby's movements and various twinges.

Insomnia

This is almost as common as tiredness, particularly during the later stages of pregnancy. Apart from your difficulty of finding a comfortable position in bed, plus the twinges and the baby's movements, you may also have to get up to empty your bladder several times during the night. There are several things you can do to make yourself feel better about the sheer discomfort in bed when you are (as they used to say) 'big with child'. The only real solution is the birth of the child. Keep your mind on this; and on the great joy your child is going to give you. Talk to your child (see Chapter 8). Get your partner to massage your abdomen, which will help to relax an active child who may also be uncomfortable. Gentle, soft music will help. Treat every physical problem as a challenge and try to direct your thoughts to the child. But, of course, don't neglect your physical needs. Plenty of pillows under the bulge or propping yourself upright can make sleep easier. Some couples find it easier at this time to sleep in separate beds, but this doesn't help the bonding process; the child is aware of both of you at this time (see Chapter 7). You should use periods when you are awake to make contact with your baby.

Stretch marks

These are believed to be caused by high levels of cortisone and progesterone and the amount of weight gained. They usually appear on the abdomen, but may also appear on breasts and thighs. The best way to prevent these is not by applying oils to the skin (which, contrary to popular belief, do not prevent stretch marks), but by being careful with your diet throughout pregnancy and avoiding too much weight gain.

Swelling

Swelling (oedema) of the feet and ankles is caused by a build-up of fluid in the body during pregnancy. There is often a pooling of fluid in the lower parts of the legs during hot weather and when you have been standing for a long time. It occurs especially at the end of the day, and often disappears in the morning. It is not in itself a serious condition, but it should be reported to your doctor or midwife. In most cases of swelling, putting your feet up is the best treatment. And always wear a pair of comfortable shoes.

Finally, remember, whatever goes wrong in pregnancy, it's your baby telling you something. By looking after yourself you are looking after your baby, attending to his needs.

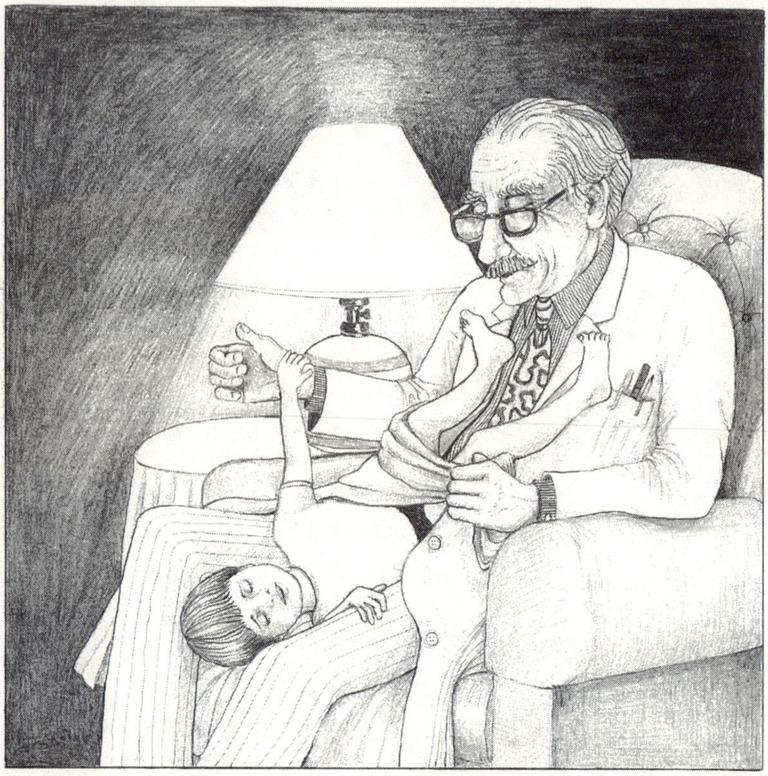

5

Birth and prenatal memories

There's a revolution going on in the way we see the world. In science and medicine today there's a movement away from authoritarianism and specialization towards a more responsible and 'holistic' way of looking at things. Tolstoy, in his great novel, *War and Peace*, anticipated the sort of science that is gaining favour today, calling it 'the science of the whole', which he said was the only true science because it explained the whole creation and the human being's place in it.

In this science everything has a function in the scheme of things, and subjective knowledge (what one knows through experience, intuition etc) is as important as objective knowledge. Objective knowledge is not the whole or the only truth, as scientists have led us to believe, because in order to acquire this kind of knowledge there must, of course, be a knowing subject. The one can't exist without the other. There is always an interplay between subject and object.

Nowadays we describe this way of looking at the world as 'holism' – spelt without the 'w' because the root of the word, from the Greek for 'whole', is related to the word 'holy'. The 'whole' is sacred, inviolate, and cannot be divided into independent, autonomous parts. For centuries we've seen the whole as split into two halves: what's inside and what's outside. In other words, subject and object, or me as I experience the world and the world that is 'out there' and is said to exist without me. What goes on inside, in the head or imagination, is subjective and therefore unpredictable and can't be measured. It can play no part in science, we've been told. Now that world-view has been turned upside down by sub-atomic physicists, who find that they can't see 'things' that could be said to exist apart from the observer. The way you look at the infinitesimally small sub-atomic world changes what you see. All one can say is that there is a two-way process: interactions between the observer and the thing observed. In other words, you see what can only be described as interactions and nothing that could be perceived as purely objective fact.

Following in Tolstoy's footsteps, a prenatal psychologist, Francis Mott, wrote a book (published in 1964) on the theme of what he called 'the universal design of creation'. Mott saw the universe as consisting of a two-way flow, like the flow of the blood through the womb, or, as he put it, having a 'paternal' focus linked by the constant back and forth flow with a 'maternal' periphery. This pattern is typical of all phenomena in the universe – from the atom to the mind. It is expressed in religion through various symbols, like the yin-yang symbol of Taoism, which shows black merging with white. In nature one sees this as light overcoming darkness or the night obliterating the day. Carl Jung described this phenomena – black, white; right, wrong; good, bad – as 'the balancing function of opposites'. Without black there wouldn't be white. Without day there wouldn't be night. Without the subject there wouldn't be an object.

Another universal rule is that nothing stands still. There is movement all the time in ourselves and in everything we see. It is a rhythmical movement that often has a sound like the heart beat, or it is silent and empty, but has boundaries, like the sea, or the sky, or the desert, and creates an atmosphere which has its own sounds – the sounds of silence – like the sounds one hears in the darkness of the night or in the heat of the day: throbbing, humming, whirring sounds, which are sometimes very loud, punctuating the silence, but at other times hardly audible.

The universal creative design

Prenatal psychologists who see life in this way – as a pulsating, to-and-fro movement, that is both seen and experienced and is going on everywhere, following a universal creative design – believe that whatever happens 'outside' affects the 'inside', and vice versa. There's no clear-cut division between outside and inside, or between mind and body. The unborn baby, they say, as he or she grows in the womb, shares the same environment with the mother and everything that goes on in the mother's world can affect the unborn child. You can't possibly look at these two beings, mother and child, at whatever stage the child has developed, as two distinct, separate beings, each going his or her own way. Neither can you look at the child as entirely dependent on the mother. There is, as in everything else, a two-way movement going on as the child grows in the womb.

The psychiatrist Dr Frank Lake believed that the unborn child was invaded by the emotional states of the pregnant mother throughout the nine months of pregnancy. He described how the mother's emotions changed the chemistry of her body which crossed over the placenta and became part of the chemistry of the unborn child. He believed that behavioural reactions of a pregnant mother affected her unborn child, including its perception of itself, through the 'cellular' memories that go on influencing our behaviour throughout life. These memories he described as 'holograms' that went on sending out their signals in every one of the body's cells. To quote his own words:

> The holograms of cellular memory are still broadcasting from infinitesimally small, but collectively transmitting stations. These minute radio stations belong to successive periods of development, from conception to implantation and the developmental stages of pregnancy. It seems they are still transmitting and it is possible to tune in to them. By these means you can distinguish what typically belongs to the first trimester (the first three months of pregnancy) or the second with its free-floating movement and what belongs to the gradual closing that occurs in the last three months before birth takes place.

These are ideas that are, for most of us, difficult to accept, because we tend to support the kind of science that has been popular for centuries (but is rapidly becoming outmoded) that sees the world as split into subject and object. We don't accept subjective evidence as having any validity unless it can be checked objectively – i.e. statistically. If it doesn't fit into any statistical pattern, it is discarded as irrelevant. So a whole lot of things that are very important in our understanding of life – things that can't be measured – are overlooked.

Most of us have memories of what happened to us at birth; but it is difficult to retrieve them – or when we do have glimpses of ourselves at the very beginning, we don't recognize them or refuse to acknowledge them.

Children's memories of birth

Children, however, who are close to the birth experience, find, with a little encouragement, no difficulty in recalling their birth. For the infant his world is simply a continuation of life in the womb.

Children in fact sometimes do strange things that can only be explained by going back to something that happened at birth. Take, for example, Rowan, who distressed her parents when she kept on pushing herself to the corner of her cot, lodging her head sharply and uncomfortably against the bars. This strange behaviour also mystified the psychiatrist Dr William Emerson until he was told by the parents that the little girl had had a long and difficult birth. The total length of labour had been eighteen hours and Rowan was stuck for the last four and a half hours. Rowan's head was crowning (ie showing at the vaginal opening) for two-and-a-half-hours and during all this time there had been a lot of pressure in a band around the top of her ears and eyebrows, where there were some broken capillaries.

Dr Emerson helps children who have had painful birth experiences by re-enacting the birth with them, usually in a playful way that doesn't distress them. He also plays music or uses massage to bring back memories, and he gets the mother or both parents to become involved in any play. It is often a lengthy procedure, but usually Dr Emerson gets to the root of a child's behavioural problem which is often to be found in some physical or emotional difficulty during pregnancy or birth.

To quote another of Dr Emerson's cases, Rory was a very difficult 14-month-old infant, who used to go into great rages and kick and scream when he was being fed. He would become very panicky when put on his back while his nappy was being changed.

His birth had been extremely traumatic. Labour began at 6 pm and continued for 22½ hours until 4.30 pm the following day. After 5 hours in hospital Rory, who had become stuck in the birth canal, was delivered by forceps. When he was born he stopped breathing and had mucus in his throat. His breathing was restored and he then spent three days in intensive care where he was fed by tubes.

Through developing appropriate games that recreated the conditions of Rory's birth, Dr Emerson, with the help of the parents, gradually removed the anxiety that led to the child's disturbed behaviour.

The two cases cited above have a fairly obvious physical cause, but there are others – according to psychotherapists who practise regression therapy – that can be traced back to emotional stress in the mother or the mother's rejection of her child during pregnancy or at birth. Take, for example, the case of a boy of five, who was a patient of the paediatrician and psychoanalyst, the late David Winnicott. In his book, *Birth Memories, Trauma and Anxiety,* Winnicott describes how the boy had been rejected by his mother and was nervous and withdrawn. Winnicott spent a lot of time with him, trying to win his confidence. The boy came repeatedly towards him and then backed away nervously. This went on for some time, but eventually the boy climbed onto Winnicott's lap. Then something rather bizarre happened. The boy got inside Winnicott's coat, turned upside down and slid down between the legs. He did this again and again. Winnicott didn't, however, say anything more about the child in his book, except that he was psychotic. Today, the child could be helped through the sort of regression therapy practised by Dr Emerson.

Of course, not all memories of birth experiences are unpleasant or related to any serious physical or emotional condition. Most births could not be described as traumatic, but small things that may pass for normal in children's dreams or play may relate to birth and could possibly point to a problem. Children, for instance, are fond of hiding, crawling under beds or under sheets; they curl up in hollows which, for instance, they sometimes dig in the sand at the seaside, and they cul up in bed, of course. They often choose the foetal position as the most comfortable one when going to sleep. This kind of behaviour obviously brings back the feelings of safety and security that they knew in the womb. On the other hand, there are children who have a horror of small, enclosed spaces or tunnels. They suffer from claustrophobia; and this may go back to some fear or anxiety during the birth process.

If you watch children at play, you are bound to see some activity that relates to the prenatal or birth experience; and it may tell you something about the child's birth and how he can suffer pain and anxiety, and how the experience of birth can shape a child's personality.

Children's dreams and nightmares also sometimes go back to the birth experience. I have a vivid memory myself of a recurring nightmare I had as a child. In the nightmare I have the sensation of everything spinning around me. It's like a whirlpool and I'm being sucked in. I'm not there. There's no me, no ego. I'm the sucking-in sensation itself. Suddenly, however, in the cataclysm, I discover a bit of myself and I try to call out to the angels to rescue me, but I find to my horror I haven't got a voice. I try and try, but no sound comes. I'm sweating, my heart is pounding . . . I can't breathe. And then it all happens. The sound barrier is broken. I scream and scream and my scream rattles the dust in the shadows and there's the sound of footsteps hurrying along the corridor outside. Mother gets into bed with me. And I cuddle up to her. I feel safe and secure again. She's there; and I'm there. I thought I'd lost her. It was like losing myself. She and I together are the whole world.

It's a childish nightmare, but it's also what you could call a memory of a memory. It's all about the terrors of a difficult birth. I was a huge baby, about 12 lb in weight – and after I was born, mother had to have some stitches to repair the damage. Deep in the roots of my being is that memory, and accompanying it is the memory of a mother's love.

A baby's cries

Babies usually cry at birth, but nobody sees this as at all distressing. In fact the mother is usually overjoyed at the sound of the baby's voice. At least the cry means the baby is alive.

But Dr David Chamberlain, a psychologist practising in San Diego, California, believes that the baby's cry is not, as is generally believed, merely reflexive, without meaning, but his re-birthing work convinces him that the infant is often distressed at birth and in pain, and he feels the pain as intensely as his cry indicates. Dr Chamberlain tells the story of his own granddaughter Bevin, who, at the age of two, was talking about her birth and asked her parents, 'Why did they poke me with a thing?' 'What thing?' her mother asked. 'Like a pencil', she said. 'They hurted me.' She was probably referring to a heel stick, an instrument for taking a sample of blood from a newborn.

Bevin is now an adult and has re-lived her birth experience under hypnosis. She had this memory of what happened to her in the delivery room:

> Now she's scooping me up from the doctor and laying me on this cold, cold, horribly hard, metal scales. It's so straight and so hard against my back. And I'm screaming because it's so painful! It hurts so much to be on this hard thing . . . I am screaming and screaming and no one is coming. Someone put something in my eyes! It's so cold; it stings, it burns . . . I'm still screaming . . . That was as hard as I could cry! It hurt . . .

Even in 1988 a medical book, *The World of the Newborn*, by D. and C. Maurer, stated that the pain of the newborn was unlike our pain. The same was once said of slaves! How doctors know the extent of a newborn's pain is not explained. In this context, a comment made by Bertrand Russell in his *Human Knowledge, its Scope and Limitations,* is apt. He relates how 'a fisherman once told me that fish have neither sense nor sensation but how he knew this he could not tell me!' Professor Liley quotes this with reference to the commonly-held belief that the baby at birth is without a sense of pain in the way we feel it. He adds: 'It would be prudent to consider at least the possibility that birth is a painful experience for a baby.'

Because of the belief that newborns didn't feel much pain, if any at all, surgeons would operate on them without an anaesthetic. In the American magazine, *Birth,* a letter (June 1986) described the barbaric practice of some surgeons in the USA who operated on premature babies with the aid of curare, a powerful drug which paralysed the child without relieving the pain.

As more and more people attend re-birthing classes, birth memories are becoming very common among children. But there are also cases of adults who are finding that they can retrieve birth memories which are medically verifiable, although in many cases they could have had no notion of what was happening in the technical sense. Psychoanalysts in the past have sometimes worked with a patient's memories of birth, notably a famous pupil of Freud, Otto Rank, who first described birth trauma.

Re-birthing techniques

Re-birthing techniques have become very sophisticated and one or other of them can be made to work for most people. Until the 1950s there were only a few psychoanalysts who believed that birth could have any influence on the development of personality. But then drug therapy began to be used for the treatment of the mentally disturbed, and psychoanalysis lost its hold. Psychiatrists began to use the drug lysergic acid diethylamide (LSD) for what is called abreactive therapy – i.e. taking a neurotic or psychotic patient back to the origin of his or her problems. When abreacting the patient experiences the past as if it were a present reality. In other words, he or she relives the past.

We know from neurological experiments that there is a part of the brain which, when stimulated by an electrode, will bring back pictures of the past. But it's not like looking at pictures in an album. What the patient sees is something like a three-dimensional movie picture, in which he or she plays the central role. The patient is both the dreamer and the dream.

LSD can do something similar, stimulating that part of the brain that takes you back to the past as if you were going through the same experiences again, only in a symbolic way: the past becomes a nightmare, a surrealist dream, which has to be interpreted.

Psychiatrists, such as Stanislav Grof in the USA and Frank Lake in the United Kingdom, got very surprising results in their LSD sessions. They expected their patients to recall events in their early childhood – this was normal – but many of them seemed to be reliving the birth experience. Frank Lake was both baffled and intrigued. He wrote:

> In 1954 people began to tell me not only the things Freud wrote about – about babies having bad disappointments at the breast and so on – they began to tell me that they were reliving their births – and they looked as though they were and I didn't know what to make of it. I wrote down everything they said and I found it difficult to accept any of it. Then I went to an

> international conference and was told that yes, people were reliving their births and it was the neurologist's job to explain how it happened.

A typical case was that of a clergyman who described how in a number of LSD sessions he went down into his 'deepest self'. It was all pain and misery and death. But 'pain let out is health let in'. In conjunction with LSD Lake gave his patient 12 mg of methadine intravenously and this precipitated a very early abreaction. The clergyman said: 'I am small, tiny and shrivelled, a small baby, a few inches in length – a little wizened baby. My mouth is dry . . . hands clammy, trembling . . .' Many hundreds of memories of this kind triggered off by LSD were reported by both Frank Lake and Stanislav Grof. Grof made a careful study of all his cases and was able to divide them into what he called Basic Perinatal Matrices (BPM). These were clusters of matrices or behaviour patterns (i.e. patterns in the adult behaviour of his clients) which correspond to the four stages of biological birth.

Basic perinatal matrices

Very briefly, BPM 1 to 4 could be described as follows:

BPM 1
The undisturbed state in the womb. The feeling of bliss, union with the mother or a feeling of rejection or of being poisoned by alcohol, tobacco or some other drug. Grof describes these two states as 'the good womb' and 'the bad womb'.

The 'good womb' can be reactivated in life by positive feelings, such as a feeling of self-esteem or of creativity or by feelings of joy in some natural setting – for instance by the sea or in a forest, walking through crisp autumn leaves – when you may have an almost mythical sense of 'oneness' which Freud called the 'oceanic' feeling.

The 'bad womb' is the opposite of this: feelings of being unloved, rejected, feelings of self-disgust and of being in a menacing or cruel environment. A fear of nature: of the sea, mountains, forests and so on.

BPM 2
The first clinical stage of delivery. This is when contractions

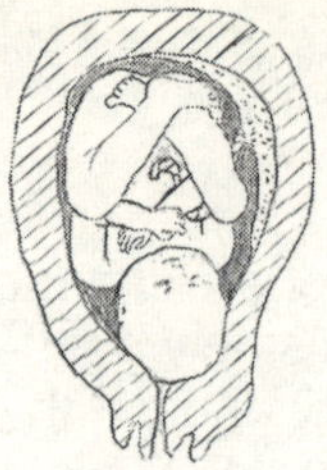

BPM 1: *The undisturbed state in the womb.*

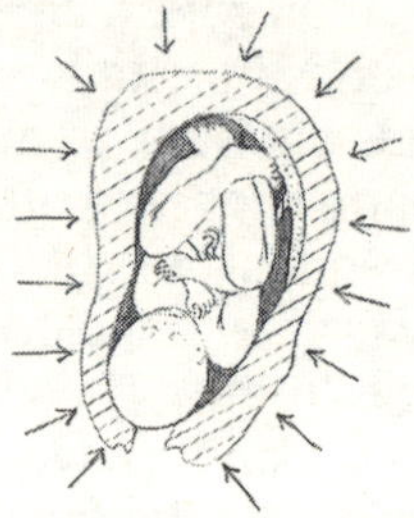

BPM 2: *The first clinical stage of delivery. Contractions take place and the child has the sensation of being stuck.*

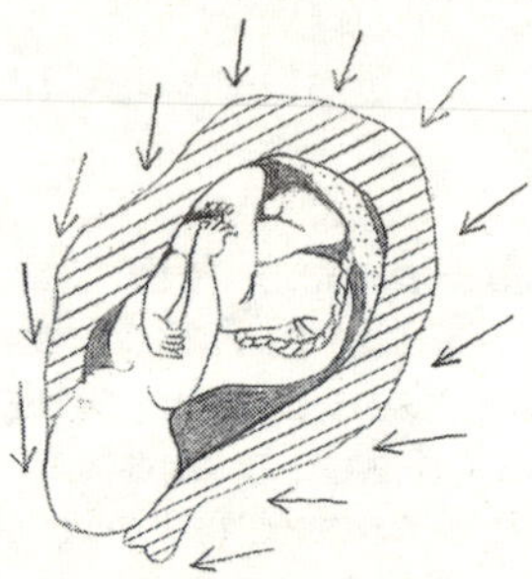

BPM 3: *Second stage of delivery. Propulsion through the birth canal.*

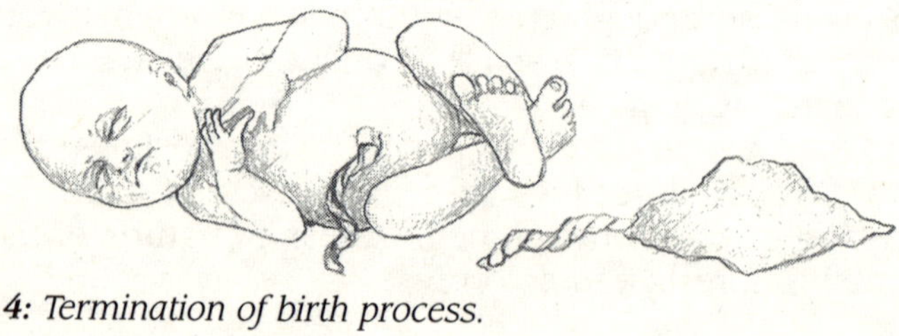

BPM 4: *Termination of birth process.*

How the biological stages of birth correspond to the Basic Preinatal Matrices

take place. The sensation for the child is one of nowhere to go or 'no exit'. There's a feeling of helplessness, maybe of panic, depending on the mother's ability to cope with the situation. Feelings of helplessness or panic may be reactivated in precarious situations, during emergencies of one sort or another – in wartime, or in a hospital ward, being anaesthetised before an operation. Calmness and control in situations like this may have their origin in a mother's self-confidence and control over her breathing during the contractions at birth.

BPM 3

The propulsion through the birth canal in the second stage of delivery is recalled in LSD sessions as a titanic struggle, at times of volcanic ecstasy. Later in life the feelings come back in battle, storms at sea, in great feats in sport or exploration – living dangerously against the elements; and also, according to Grof, in highly sensual activities: sexual orgies and the like. Lake describes the essential movement of the unborn child during this stage as a vigorous forward and backward thrust of the pelvis. 'If this adult function is paralysed by unknown fears,' says Lake, 'it is to the second stage of delivery that we must look for the pathological link-up and therefore the therapeutic key.'

BPM 4

The termination of the birth process and of the events in the third clinical stage of delivery is recalled in LSD sessions as an expansion of space, visions of gigantic halls, radiant light and beautiful colour. The feelings of birth are reactivated in many different ways: as anxiety when changing from one condition to another – e.g. a change of lifestyle – a sensation of elation or one of fear when looking down from a great height.

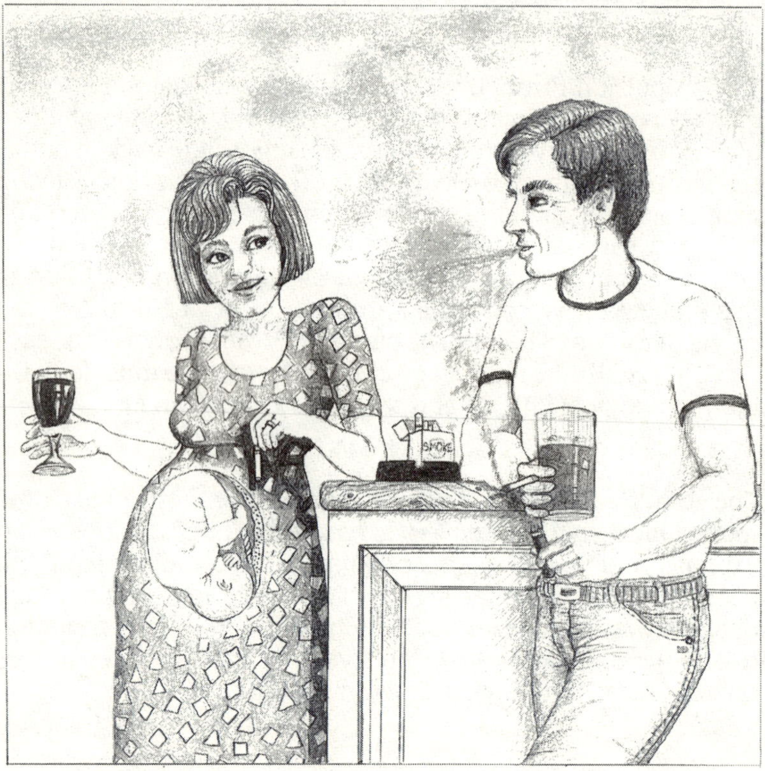
SMOKE

6

Preventing and healing prenatal wounds

Research work on drug-induced states of mind, which triggered off birth memories, came to an end in the late 1960s when LSD was banned both in the USA and the United Kingdom. But something much more exciting and less harmful took its place. Frank Lake was one of those who discovered that you didn't need drugs to bring back prenatal and birth memories. There were other simpler methods, including Reichian deep breathing and guided fantasy. For this you just needed a guide or facilitator to help you recover your memories. The guide would help you to reproduce – in the imagination – the process of prenatal growth and birth. Lake called this 'contextualizing' the process: i.e. reproducing the 'feeling context' of being enclosed or of lying deep in a cavern, or any other kind of symbolic womb that could be used in a guided fantasy. Or games could be played to reproduce the struggle of birth during the various stages of delivery mentioned in the last chapter. You begin with a fantasy, but after a while the reality supervenes. More of this later.

The psychoanalysts had demonstrated the ease with which some patients could abreact through free association. And hypnosis had also been used to help a patient to recover early memories.

The psychoanalysts had discovered that in most of us there was a censor at work, in what they termed the subconscious, blocking unpleasant thoughts and feelings associated with very early traumatic experiences. Bringing back the memories helped to release you from the pain. But classical psychoanalysis did not attempt to bring back birth memories, and the process of helping a patient to overcome neurotic symptoms was often long and painful.

What Lake and his followers discovered was that there was a sort of undercover agent (or guardian angel, if you like) working for us, not only against us, as the Freudian censor does, all the time. Some of your memories are indeed blocked; but you will find that by getting in touch with yourself, your true self, as distinct from the self-image – by going down and down into the depths – you don't meet what many people are afraid of meeting, namely, some kind of primordial beast or the animal impulses lurking there. On the contrary, you find there's a lot of energy and a lot of joy and a lot of love waiting to be released. 'There is no beast in man,' said Carl Rogers. 'There is only man in man.'

It's not the Freudian censor who stands in your way. It's usually 'what people think', or 'what others say', and, for the normally-educated and conforming sort of person, it's what Science says, that stands in the way. Science will not allow anything to exist that cannot be measured or put into some kind of category. As R. D. Laing says, there are certain experiences that have no place in the scheme of things because the scheme of things has no place for the experiences. That's how it is. An impasse! So, for fear of being ridiculed, you disown feelings within yourself that you know perfectly well are there. You block them off. Then what you need most of all is a helping, friendly hand – a hand stretched out to the child in you, with its offer of freedom to be yourself.

Many of us have memories that go way back, sometimes before conception: collective memories or family memories that go on bothering people for generation after generation – and we don't know what it is that is causing us so much pain. A whole race of people can suffer in this way from some trauma that goes back to the distant historical past. All these memories are pre-verbal. Whether they are passed down or not, they go back to a time when you didn't have any words, when you were a child, or were still in the womb waiting to be born – so the memories were recorded, not in the cognitive centres of the brain, but more in the sensory network of nerves and cells and they come back as feelings, or tastes or sounds or scents. We all have these memories. In my own case, early memories are triggered off by the smell of honeysuckle or of hot tar bubbling up between the cracks in paving stones on a summer's day. An early memory, which, however, is indistinct, comes back to me as a taste of something I cannot quite identify that's sweet and a bit like milk. It could be a memory of my mother's milk – but I don't know. There are all kinds of sensations that can act as triggers. A movement, particularly a rocking movement, can trigger a memory. Many of our pleasures, like dancing to the rhythm of a pulsating kind of music, like the beat of the heart, or in childhood the fairground swings and roundabouts will recall the movement you so often felt in the womb.

There's a story told by the French dramatist and critic Jean Cocteau in his diary about going back to his boyhood home in 1953. He was interested to see if by going back he could recover some of the feelings he had when he lived there. Could he relive his childhood or parts of it?

Unfortunately, the man who lived in his old home wouldn't let him in. Cocteau looked round at the street and the houses and found everything had changed; and he wondered if it was at all possible to bring back his childhood memories without going into the house.

Cocteau then recalled that as a child he would walk close to the houses in the road and trail his finger along the wall. He did this again, hoping that memories would come flooding back. But they didn't. There were a few memories, but they were thin and pale.

Suddenly, he remembered that as a child his hand had trailed along the wall at a different level. He was, of course, much smaller at that time. So, bending down and closing his eyes, he again moved his finger along the wall. The result was remarkable:

> Just as the needle picks up the melody of the record, I obtained the melody of the past with my hand. I found everything: my cape, the leather of my satchel, the names of my friends and of my teachers, certain expressions I had used, the sound of my grandfather's voice, the smell of his beard, the smell of my sister's dresses, and of my mother's gown.

Getting to know the child in you

All couples should become aware, by their own experiments, of their own beginnings if they are planning to become parents.

For them, the object of 're-birthing' is not only to heal the wounds that may have been inflicted on them in childhood, but to bring back the memory of what it means to be a child; and I am referring here not only to the visible child after birth, but to the child before birth: he's the same person. For so many of us that child simply doesn't exist. We have lost touch with our beginnings – with the child in us. As we grew up we were taught 'to put away childish things'. We were taught that children were 'silly', 'irresponsible', 'stupid', 'immature'. So we rejected the child in us. We rejected all the good things – being spontaneous, creative, free, trusting, loving and so on. We threw away the baby with the bath water!

Frank Lake would use what he called the deep-sea fantasy to help someone to bring back prenatal memories. Taking his client in the imagination to some deep cave in the sea set the tone of the session, giving it a feeling context. 'The person lying relaxed on the floor', said Dr Lake, 'as he visualizes his watery descent will suddenly begin to pick up primal images, very faint at first, but becoming stronger and stronger.'

Lake also used Reichian deep breathing. The way this works is as follows: the client is told to 'breathe up into your strength. Wait . . . Now down into your weakness (or whatever else emerges of primal joy or grief). Wait . . . Now up again . . .' As you breathe out you make a deep sound resonating downwards. You take the stream of attention down into your belly and observe what is coming in – and, whatever it is, good or bad, you give it a voice.

At that particular moment someone might say: 'This is beautiful. She's so warm. She doesn't know I'm here, but she's such a loving, warm person.' Someone else might say: 'It's very cold in here.'

The words, of course, are not the memory. It is the adult talking, trying to express the feelings that come to the surface during the exercise. The unborn baby is given a voice by the adult as he picks up primal feelings of warmth or frigidity. Connections are made between early physical feelings and later emotional states – it's *warm:* I feel loved: it's *cold:* I feel unloved, rejected. The adult does the talking; and behind the talk the unborn child is there afraid, unloved, inarticulate, just a sound – which may break out in the course of a session – a scream in the darkness.

Maternal emotions and foetal activity

I mentioned in an earlier chapter how maternal emotions affect the unborn child. Research is a bit ragged, but at least it can be said that such research as there is shows conclusively that there is always increased foetal activity (the hyperactive foetus) at times when mothers are under severe emotional stress or suffer chronic anxiety during pregnancy.

No one can be certain of the long-term effects of hyperactivity in the foetus; but there is growing interest in prenatal determinants of personality and a great deal of research is at present going on in this area in the USA and in Europe. Professor Van Den Bergh, of the Department of Psychology, University of Leuven, Belgium, has carried out some very careful experiments to measure maternal emotions and their effect on foetal behaviour. His subjects were ten fairly normal healthy women, between the ages of 19 and 31 with durations of pregnancy of between 36 and 40 weeks.

The anxiety state of the mother was measured according to an accepted tool of measurement called the State-Trait Anxiety Inventory, which can differentiate between an anxiety state that reflects current tension or apprehension and is fluctuating, and what is called 'trait' anxiety, which is a person's disposition or proneness to anxiety in many situations. The unborn child's behaviour was recorded by ultrasound (echograph recording) and measuring the foetal heart beat. Emotions were induced in the mother by showing a film of a normal birth. This is not likely to get the pulse racing as in some situations which one could imagine; but it was of intense interest to the mother and would probably induce the normal anxiety of a pregnant woman, who for the first time was watching the procedures of childbirth.

If something as relatively mild as this could change the behaviour of the unborn child, then a severe emotional disturbance would probably have a very profound effect on the child. Van Den Bergh did, in fact, find a significant correlation between the mother's emotional state (expressed medically as 'mean state anxiety') at those moments when an echograph recording was being made and the child's activity. The film itself didn't seem to have any observable maternal emotional effect that could be said to produce a change in foetal behaviour. It's interesting that it was the technology that upset the mother and child.

Some follow-up research (published in 1988) confirmed these findings, but it also revealed that a chronic state of anxiety during pregnancy produced marked changes in foetal behaviour and activity. One interesting outcome of the research, as Van Den Bergh points out in his report, is the possibility that ultrasound could have a 'biofeedback' effect on the mother, which would lower anxiety states. If you see your 'anxiety' or the effect of it recorded on a screen, you can control it; there's an unconscious, or what some call a passive process of control, which is how biofeedback works.

A more drastic and rather cruel experiment was carried out by the Austrian obstetrician, Emil Reinhold, to establish the speed with which a mother's sudden feeling of alarm registered on the unborn child. What Dr Reinhold did was to place a number of women in a relaxed position under an ultrasound machine. What he didn't tell them was that when they were lying in this position the unborn child would also be perfectly relaxed. He then told the mother that her baby wasn't moving. This immediately alarmed the mother and within a matter of seconds the unborn baby was kicking furiously.

It has been established that maternal smoking can damage the unborn child physically, but there is also some evidence that when a pregnant woman merely starts smoking the unborn child becomes alarmed. A remarkable study carried out by Michael Lieberman in 1970 and published in the *American Journal of Obstetrics* showed that when the mother was thinking about putting a cigarette to her lips, the foetal heart rate went up. Presumably, in this case, the desire to smoke was brought on by some feeling of nervousness or anxiety and this was communicated to the unborn child.

The bereaved mother

It is fairly well-established that there is a relationship between the mother's anxiety and the unborn child's activity which increases according to the intensity of the mother's feelings of apprehension. But what of the other emotions, such as sorrow or joy? Empirical studies of thousands of people who have taken part in re-birthing sessions show that the unborn child is sensitive to a wide range of emotions, including positive feelings of love, on which he naturally thrives.

There is some evidence that a bereaved mother can disturb her unborn child. I have the experience myself of having been influenced by a bereavement in the family just before I was born. I cannot say for certain that I was affected in this way in the womb, but I can trace much of what has happened to me in my life, including the way my personality developed in childhood, to the fact that my mother's father died shortly before I was born. I was a distraction and took my grandfather's place in my mother's affections. I grew up feeling that I could always comfort my mother whenever she was distressed, and this feeling, which almost amounted to a need, extended to others who were close to me. Throughout my life I've always been aware of death and have never been afraid to get close to people who were dying: in fact, I've felt almost impelled to move towards the sick and the dying and to do everything I possibly can for them. It's as if my mission in life was the conquest of death. An impossible mission!

Frank Lake describes this sort of person, who is born to a woman who suffers a loss of someone close and dear to her during pregnancy, as a 'foetal therapist'. Such a person has also been described as suffering from 'the rescuer syndrome'. Later in life he or she tends to look for work in the healing professions.

Lake's theory was that a pregnant woman's distress resulted in what he called 'the negative umbilical "affect"' (i.e. the displacement of feelings). The mother's feelings of distress would cross the placenta; the unborn child would then try to push the feelings away and would be displaced and finish up in some part of the body – the skin, eyes, or feet or any other part of the body – which Lake believed accounted for many psychosomatic illnesses. There's no hard evidence for this; but Lake had many patients whom he said had strange physical problems which were chronic and baffled doctors, but were cured when their origin was traced to some maternal emotional disturbance that affected the unborn child.

He described a woman whose negative umbilical affect went into her feet. The woman, who was a nursing sister on an obstetrics ward, consulted Dr Lake because, for no accountable reason, she was constantly ripping skin off her feet.

'When she went into this,' said Dr Lake, 'she said, "I don't understand. My mother loves me. She has always loved me." She was convulsed with weeping as she pushed all the "badness" into her feet. She's always felt that her thighs were ugly, and heavy and painful, but as a matter of fact she's got beautiful shapely thighs.'

Symbolically, Dr Lake said, she was carrying all the distress from the umbilical input.

'But what was this weeping for?' asked Dr Lake. 'She couldn't believe that her mother could be responsible for it'.

Then she recalled that three months before she was conceived her grandfather – her mother's father – was diagnosed as suffering from an incurable cancer. The mother nursed him throughout his illness until he died at the end of the first three months of pregnancy. The unborn child was invaded by the mother's grief; hence the weeping, the sadness that was pushed into the feet.

Lessons

The lessons are obvious. Prenatal and birth memories are all saying one thing, loud and clear – namely, that the child is the product, emotionally and physically, of the parents' way of being, which we call lifestyle. 'Style' is all important: and this means your style in relation not only to what you eat and how you live and where you live, but also to what you think and how you feel. This style may go back for centuries – and there may be a blemish, like a black thread running through a family's pattern of behaviour which goes on repeating itself from one generation to the next.

The British surgeon and psychiatrist, Dr Kenneth McCall, has written a fascinating account of his technique of healing supposedly 'incurable' patients whom he believes are victims of ancestral control. He liberates them from this control by drawing up a Family Tree in which the ancestor who was causing the patient harm is identified. He then cuts the bond between the ancestor and the patient by celebrating, with a clergyman, a service of Holy Communion which delivers the tormented ancestor to God. In his book, *Healing the Family Tree* (Sheldon Press, London, 1985), Dr McCall describes many of his successful cases. For many, this kind of treatment may be unacceptable, but there are many who are bothered, in one way or another, by the ghosts of their ancestors; and for some, exorcism (which in effect is what McCall is doing) has been shown to work.

But as far as most pre-birth and birth memories are concerned, they not only help those who suffer from some traumatic experience at or before birth, they can also help in preventing a repetition of a family pattern that may not go back very far. Dr Emerson is often asked by parents whether birth can cause lifelong changes in personality and behaviour. He says the answer is both yes and no, depending on the degree of impact, and whether the impact occurs depends on several factors:

1. The extent of trauma or difficulty around the birth itself.
2. The degree to which life experiences continue to support or reinforce the birth experience.
3. The quality of prenatal emotional and physical care, especially nutrition.
4. The quality of maternal and paternal infant bonding.

Positive feelings for the child will overcome the difficulties a child may encounter at birth. Even before birth the bonding process depends on the mother's love for the child. It can more than offset the anxieties and stresses that are normal occurrences in everybody's life.

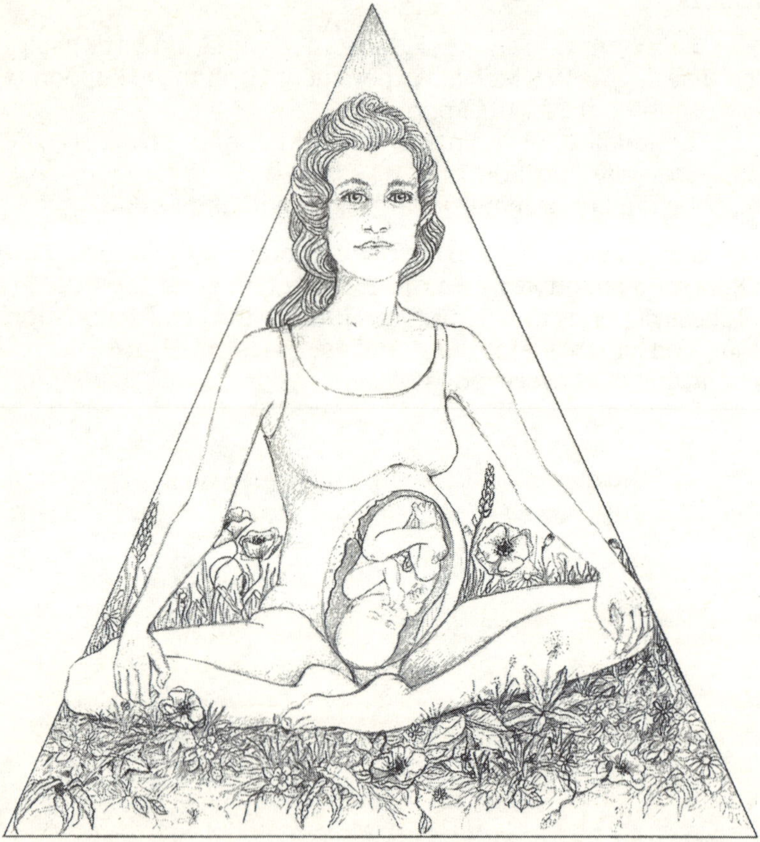

7

Prenatal bonding

You are handed your baby, or should be handed your baby immediately after birth, and though you feel exhausted, you will go through certain rituals which are common to most mothers. You will start with fingertip touching of hands and feet and proceed in four to eight minutes to massaging and stroking the whole body with the palms of the hands.

The mother always shows an intense interest in the baby's eyes. It is important for her to see the eyes and to make eye-to-eye contact with her baby as soon as possible. Often when the baby's eyes are closed in sleep the mother will wake up the baby so that they can both enjoy the intimate personal relationship of eye-to-eye contact. The baby doesn't mind being aroused. He enjoys being gazed at by his mother; and he will return her gaze with equal intensity.

These interactions in the first few minutes and hours of life are known as bonding and are recognized now as being very important in the healthy development of the baby's personality and sense of confidence in his environment. But, important though it is, this is not the beginning of the bonding process. What we are witnessing is the start of the important visual interactions combined with all the others, but as a matter of fact, a lot has gone on before birth that enables the child to interact with his mother. The bonding at birth is the culmination of a process which has been going on since conception. The strength of the bond depends on the way the mother has looked after herself and her baby before birth. And, it should be said, both parents are involved in this. The man plays an important role in the bonding process.

Bonding is a fairly new concept, dating back to the 1960s

when it was first realized that there was a form of communication which brought a mother and child closely together after birth. They recognized each other at the moment of birth and an attachment developed between them. It's been known for a very long time, of course, that something like this goes on in nature. You see it happening everywhere in the animal world. For instance, in the thousands of pairing birds that have their nests packed closely together on rocks near the sea, each couple forms a close attachment to its own brood immediately after birth, and it's obvious that parents and chicks communicate in various ways, through sight, sound and smell. It's amazing how among all those thousands of birds, all looking exactly alike, each couple can pick out its own offspring – each pair has a powerful biological urge to protect and feed their young. The survival of a species depends to a large extent on the development of this close bond between parents and offspring.

Bonding in humans is similar: it's a two-way process in which mother and child form a close attachment. The process has been studied in primates – for instance, in the well-known work of Harry and Margaret Harlow at the University of Wisconsin. What their work showed was that touch, and the softness or texture of what is touched, were important in developing a sense of belonging and a feeling of safety and trust between a mother and child.

Everybody knows the feeling of cuddliness or lovableness in a child or even a baby animal and how compelling it can be. You have a strong urge to pick it up and stroke it and hold it close to you. It's the way the young survive. The human infant, however, may object to anyone but his own mother picking him up and cuddling him. He may feel threatened by the attentions of strangers. He recognizes the feel and smell and sound of his own mother. It all adds up to a feeling of belonging, a feeling of safety. We all have that feeling at birth. It's a feeling that never really leaves us. Bonding is as real as the smell of fresh air or the taste of strawberries. It runs like a thread through all our senses and extends outwards from the early sense of closeness to a mother to the sense of closeness that develops for others.

The strength of the bond with your mother comes back to you later in life with the birth of your own child. If the bond was strong between you and your own mother, the likelihood is that you will develop a strong bond with your own children. If, on the other hand, your mother rejected you, it is quite probable that you will reject your own children unless you can repair the damage that your mother did to you and maybe that her mother did to her. The problem may go back many generations.

The Harlows found that a sense of belonging can, amazingly, be developed in monkeys for an inanimate object, if it can provide them with milk. As I said, the Harlows demonstrated that in forming this bond, a sense of touch was important. They took a group of monkeys away from their mothers immediately after birth (which, even in the interests of science, seems a bit cruel to me) and put them in two separate cages with two different types of artificial surrogate mothers. One had a wire-framed body, a wooden head, and a wooden nipple protruding from one of its wire breasts, which supplied milk. The other was a similar contraption, but it had a terrycloth towel draped around it, with a nipple protruding through a hole in the towel.

It was found that the monkeys fed by both types of surrogate mothers drank on average the same amount of milk and gained the same weight. But when the monkeys were put in a cage with both types of surrogate mother they showed a distinct preference for the one with the terrycloth towel. They clung to her and hugged her as they would a real mother. The Harlows tell the story of how they put a tiny wind-up mechanical toy into the cage and when it clattered noisily across the floor it sent the monkeys running to the terrycloth mother. The feel of the terrycloth had given them a sense of safety as if there was a live mother there to protect them.

The sense of touch, the first sense to develop in the womb, is very powerful and important both before and after birth. In his poem *Song of Myself,* Walt Whitman talks about touch 'quivering me to a new identity'. And this is precisely what happens to the child. He gradually develops a sense of identity through touch. This sense of identity means a sense of oneness with someone else – in the first place, with a mother – and a feeling of confidence in yourself arising out of a feeling of confidence and trust in a mother. That is what happens in the bonding process. In the moments immediately after birth, when a child is at its most vulnerable, it is important to restore his confidence in his mother and reinforce the bonding process which has been going on before birth. That is why it is so important for the child and mother to be in contact immediately after birth. Quite apart from the psychological importance of this closeness, the suckling reflex is at its height twenty to thirty minutes after birth and if not satisfied will diminish, not to return again for forty hours.

Bonding starts a long time before birth. It is a process that happens naturally among primitive people because of the sort of lives they live, but in industrialized societies there are all sorts of needs, such as the need for a mother to go out to work to make money to help to pay the mortgage, which are not natural and interfere with the bonding process: so the child is not always given all the care and attention he usually gets in less industrialized societies.

The African mother is much closer to her child, both before and after birth. She is much more aware of what is going on. The bonding process is very strong and as a result of this the child becomes much more alert in his environment.

The table below shows the progress of an infant in an African family compared with the Western baby:

	Western baby	*African baby*
Holds up head	3 months	4-6 weeks
Sits up without support	7-8 months	4 months
Stands up and walks	12-14 months	8 months
Learns to run	24 months	12-14 months

Bonding is a combination of different factors; the most important, from a purely psychological point of view, is a cultural one. Our social and cultural environments impinge on the psychological and physical development of the unborn child and also on the infant in his early formative years. The loyalty a couple may have for their own particular culture or social or religious groups will have a profound influence on their lives. From the beginning their cultural background will influence their attitude to their child and to the way they bring him up, even to the extent of deciding what food they give him, which can, of course, affect his health. Even though this loyalty to one's own culture is not so strong as it used to be, cultural attitudes and customs die hard; they remain a part of one's psyche.

Confusions in today's society

Many parents in today's world lack the certainties their counterparts had in former times. For one thing, the spiritual dimension is often missing. There are no spiritual models that the majority of people find at all convincing. We have lost touch with our gods and our ideals. People no longer dream of perfection. There's no goal of perfection to work towards, no light at the end of the tunnel. For many, it's all gloom, gloom, gloom.

Although perhaps it is unrealistic to believe perfection is an attainable goal, we all like to believe in a guardian angel and a God we can turn to in times of trouble. 'God is real', said William James, 'because he produces real effects.'

There are no myths or legends that people can remember any more and relate to their children; no fireside stories. All cultures throughout history have had their myths and legends which, as Jung believed, expressed in symbolic form certain important aspects of the deep unconscious. They are aspects that relate to the very origin of life and should therefore have much to tell us about our prenatal development. But we have cut that cord, have separated ourselves from our source of being.

People in today's highly industrialized world do not realize that they are cutting themselves off from an incredibly rich source of psychological and spiritual strength. Namely, the imagination! We are into cars and videos and microwave ovens and all kinds of mechanical and electronic things. But it was dreams which created these things in the first place (i.e. the dreams of scientists) and dreams – as demonstrated by visualization techniques used, for instance, in the treatment of cancer – can heal wounds; and they can also improve interpersonal relationships and create a more harmonious environment in which to live.

Putting your dreams on paper

Some parents are not at all sure that, for one reason or another, they want children; and some only have children because of the pressures put on them by others to start a family: e.g. to provide grandchildren for their own parents and carry on the family name. For some, children are a nuisance, preventing a woman, for instance, from pursuing her career, restricting a couple's freedom and creating financial problems, because having a baby can be a very expensive business these days.

If you are in any doubt about whether you want a baby, or if you only have a baby in order to please someone else, you are already laying up trouble for yourself and your child. A strong desire or longing, shared by both partners, to have a child is an important step in the bonding process. A planned pregnancy is much more likely to produce a strong bond between parents and offspring than an unplanned one that just happens and takes you by surprise. So the first thing to do in the bonding process is to plan the family. Articulate your plans. Put your dreams on paper.

The crying baby

Any kind of stress, if it goes on too long during pregnancy, will interfere with the bonding process and will create unhappiness – or at least physical discomfort in the unborn child, who will become an inconsolable crying baby after birth.

Stress produces negative bonding (disbonding) between mother and child. The stress chemicals, including the hormone epinephrine (also known as adrenaline) are carried by the mother's bloodstream through the umbilical cord to the unborn child, causing an increase of metabolism, heartbeat and movement. Research among parents who have turbulent emotional pressures during pregnancy shows that they tend to give birth to highly irritable children, who may also have physical problems.

Sheila Kitzinger, in her book *The Crying Baby* (Viking, 1989), came to a similar conclusion. Her research, based on 14,000 questionnaires and a great many interviews, pointed to stresses in pregnancy and childbirth as the main reason for the crying baby.

A great deal of the stress in the women she questioned was caused by major life changes. For instance, one study showed that 40 per cent of women moved house during pregnancy or within six weeks of birth or were still in the throes of major alterations at that time.

One couple with a distressed baby had had constant quarrels until they separated when the wife was six-and-a-half months pregnant. They tried living together again one month later, but the quarrels broke out again and the husband assaulted his wife. They were living in poverty and had run up massive debts.

Sheila Kitzinger also describes another woman who had nursed her father through lung cancer until his death when she was eight months pregnant. The experiences quoted in this book read like some of the experiences described in re-birthing sessions. There is so much evidence now to show that prenatal experiences can have a profound effect on the later development of the child. It has been suggested that the person with a schizoid personality, who recoils from any physical stimulation, and may not like being touched, could have been over-stimulated before birth and learnt to cut off when the over-stimulated body burnt up the food and oxygen supply needed for growth.

Prebirth bonding programme

If a couple starts with a planned pregnancy in which both make the decision together, and continue with this positive approach throughout the nine months of pregnancy, sharing their experiences together and directing many of their thoughts towards the baby, tensions will be reduced, and it's unlikely any harm will be done to the baby. You won't have a crying baby on your hands.

All couples would benefit from relaxation exercises, including meditation, massage, autogenic training and biofeedback. (See resource section at end of book.) Intensive therapy should be avoided during pregnancy, such as body-oriented therapies, and primai integration including re-birthing. These therapies may be useful before and after pregnancy, but more gentle therapies are called for during pregnancy. Assertiveness training should certainly be learnt at some time before pregnancy: it is a skill you will probably need, because the pregnant woman is so vulnerable and may find it difficult to say no, particularly to a forceful midwife or male obstetrician, and this could be stressful.

You should not, however, expect to get through pregnancy without any stress. There will be difficult times, and possibly quarrels. All you have to do when arguments start building up into a flaming row is to say to each other, loud and clear, 'STOP!

THINK OF THE BABY!' But that won't always work. Rows happen. Don't brood on them. Put them behind you and try to keep the baby constantly in mind. Thinking of the baby as someone real from the start can work wonders. It can bring you together and protect the baby from any injury.

Ten-step programme of bonding

The American psychotherapist Eve Bowen, in her book *Prebirth Bonding*, (Headstart Lovestart Publications, San Diego, 1985), gives a ten-step programme of bonding, which would benefit every couple and, barring genetic and chromosomal accidents, should produce a bright and healthy baby perfectly in tune with his environment. I have incorporated some of my own comments, adaptations and additional suggestions in the Eve Bowen programme:

Step 1: rest and relaxation

You can't be good to your baby if you're not good to yourself; so both of you, mother and father, should set aside a quiet time of the day, every day, when you can rest and relax together. The months of carrying the baby will produce all kinds of swings of mood. There will be times when you simply hate being pregnant; but there will be other times when you feel on top of the world. It is important to find some space in your busy day where you can both enjoy just being together with the baby. Use this time for being quiet together, not for talking or doing anything active; and make sure you are not interrupted. 'It is surprising', says Eve, 'how many couples do not regularly set up this quiet time together, just in the normal course of their marriage. This is a wonderful time to get into the habit, a habit that could serve your partnership long after your baby is born.' You need not spend a long time together – it can be as short as ten minutes. The quality of the quiet time is more important than the number of minutes spent together. You can assess the quality by the sounds that punctuate the silence; the distant barking of a dog somewhere outside, the sound of birdsong, children's voices. Or they could be internal sounds: the beating of the heart, the sound of breathing. No thought should obstruct the sounds. They should come and go; and in between there will be total silence. The silence you aim to achieve is an extension of what happens between two thoughts.

Step 2: enjoy the baby

A week or two later, after mother and father have become used to simply being together, with nothing to do and nothing to say. Here you begin to verbalize your feelings, to talk about the baby, the coming months, the plans, the hopes and dreams. It is important to be open and honest with each other. Express all your feelings in words. Keep nothing to yourself. Approach a problem from every angle. Don't both talk at once: give the other enough time and space to have his or her say. As in co-counselling, there should be one of you just listening and not making any judgement, while the other is talking. You will find you will want to say a lot about the baby and how it is going to affect your life. It is astonishing how many couples do not share their feelings about the baby until just before (and in some cases, after) the baby arrives. Clear the air now, if indeed there is anything to clear away. Enjoy the baby. Plan how the room will look and where the baby will sleep. Begin thinking about names. Set up a positive, loving attitude for the months ahead.

Step 3: make contact with the baby

You can begin to make contact with the baby about 30-40 days after conception when the baby's heart has formed and is beating. This step, like step one, is mental. It involves your thoughts only. Direct your thoughts towards the baby. Visualize the baby as an intelligent being: sensitive, responsive, and appreciative. Send thoughts that communicate your love for the baby; let the baby know that he is coming into a loving, caring environment. Although the baby is at a very early stage of development, and will not be aware of his surroundings, let alone your presence, his inclusion in your thoughts will have a chemical effect on the mother's body and infuse the growing child with feelings of love. This might sound romantic and unreal, but that's how loving relationships do actually develop. There is a chemistry of love which our thoughts can nourish. So imagine all the time you are directing your thoughts towards the baby that you are feeding him with love.

Remember that this is your initial contact, or 'bonding': so say 'hello' in a way that you would if you wanted to make anyone you loved welcome in your life. You should add music to your rest period in step 3. Choose some music you both enjoy – not too strident. If classical music is to your taste, it has been found that the unborn child, at a later stage of development, prefers Vivaldi, Bach or Mozart to Beethoven. The music should fit your mood. It shouldn't be too obtrusive. Don't be at all surprised if, after the baby is born, it falls asleep immediately after you turn on the same music you played during these rest periods when your thoughts were being directed to your baby.

Eve Bowen suggests that both parents should rest a hand on the baby. You will, she says, feel the sensation of new life long before the baby starts kicking. And at a later stage the baby will be able to feel you. You will be able to feel the baby moving towards your hands.

The loving, welcome thoughts – to which you have added music and touch – complete the bond.

Step 4: begin to talk to your baby

The next step is to speak out loud to your baby. You may feel a bit silly doing this, but it has been shown that the sound of words are picked up by the baby and can be remembered after birth. Not the meaning, but the sound. For instance, in an experiment carried out in 1983 by a research team led by Dr Anthony Casper at the University of North Carolina, USA, it was demonstrated that a newborn child could remember words spoken to him during the last six-and-a-half weeks of pregnancy. It was a very careful scientific investigation which proved beyond any shadow of doubt that the unborn baby picked up the sound, if not the sense, of words spoken to him in the later stage of pregnancy.

The story is told in the American medical magazine *Hippocrates* of how a colleague of Dr Casper's, the psychologist Melanie Spence, attended classrooms for expectant mothers at Moses Cone Hospital. 'I am looking for pregnant women who would be willing to sit in a quiet place twice a day and read a story aloud to their unborn child', she told each group. The request brought smiles of disbelief to some and shakes of the head to many. But in the end Spence got together a team of recruits, who were asked to read portions of three stories into a tape recorder: Dr Seuss' *The Cat in the Hat,* and *The Dog and the Fog,* and *The King, the Mice and the Cheese* by Nancy and Eric Gurney.

The mothers taking part in the experiment selected a story to read to their baby. The sixteen babies tested each heard their story 67 times. Then after birth all the stories were read to the babies and it was discovered that every one without exception preferred the story that had been read to them while they were in the womb.

The way preferences were recorded was quite ingenious. It is not possible to describe the experiment in any great detail here, but basically what happened was that a rubber nipple was wired up to a tape recorder and the baby controlled what he heard by altering his sucking patterns. If he didn't like the story that was being read to him, he simply stopped sucking. The baby got the hang of it very quickly; and it was found that he sucked enthusiastically when he heard the story he'd heard so often in the womb.

So there's no doubt that reading or talking to a baby will make an impression and help the bonding process. The talk should not be too heavy. A joke would not be out of place at times. If both parents speak to the unborn baby, whatever else happens, the fact that they are speaking out loud will help to establish the threesome. Obviously, your words will let your partner know what communications you are sending, allowing him or her to join in a three-way communication.

'You are building a family here', says Eve Bowen. 'You are putting the first building blocks into place in a system of three-way communication which will serve you for years to come. Talking to your unborn baby is hardly a waste of time. Not talking to him would be the waste.'

Step 5: share your whole life

With this step, we increase the amount of time we spend with the baby. The baby becomes integrated into our life, and that means into everything we do. Jean Liedhoff, in her book *The Continuum Concept* (Penguin, 1986), describes how in non-industrialized communities the child shares the parents' interests and is not excluded from any activity. Life is a 'continuum', one activity merging with another from conception to death, and the family remain together throughout the journey, sharing their work, their joys and sorrows, their hopes and fears. This is what bonding is all about. It is the beginning of the 'continuum': it sets a pattern that is continued throughout life. It is important to experience this feeling of the whole family being together, sharing their activities, right at the beginning: it will then be easy to carry on after the child is born.

Step 6: visualization

This step puts you in touch with the deepest part of yourself where the creative process takes place, where you plan your life, where your wishes are given a shape.

Begin planning the way you want to have your baby. Draw specific images on the chalkboard of your mind. Or you could imagine a huge movie screen and project images onto it of your child's birth. Do this systematically every day. At the same time, keep up with stages 1-5.

Step 7: education

To give your visualization an authentic touch, make sure you know the medical details of pregnancy and birth and the various kinds of birth on offer. Attend antenatal classes and, if possible, go to classes for couples, not just for the pregnant woman. Remember this is a joint enterprise. The unborn baby has two parents: he doesn't want to spend most of his time with only one parent. Buy tape cassettes and video programmes. Look out for informative articles in the newspapers and magazines, including the health magazines. Talk to other pregnant women and couples, your doctor, midwife and anyone else you think may have something to contribute. Pay as much attention to educating yourself about your baby as you would to a new home you are going to buy. Become an expert on new and healthier approaches to childbirth and tell other people about how you are concentrating on your baby, caring for him and treating him as a human being from the moment you know you are pregnant. Talking to people about what you are doing will help you to keep the programme going.

Step 8: preparation

You now take the momentous step of actually preparing for the birth of your baby. Continue to do all the other things – don't stop the rest periods; keep playing music; and keep communicating with your baby. But now you must begin making lists. Try to think of everything. Discuss it all with your partner. Go over your lists again and again to make sure you haven't missed anything.

Step 9: materialization

Now, put the plans into action. Prepare a written agreement with the help of your partner. Then get your doctor to sign. Make sure that he or she and the hospital and midwife, obstetrician, whoever is concerned with your birth, fully understands it. *Insist* on getting things done your way, so long as you are sure there is no risk. This is where assertiveness training will come in useful. Talk to relatives. Often they can be persuaded to do some of the chores, leaving you and your partner to enjoy the birth together. Make sure they know when the baby is expected so that they can keep that time free. Many families make more detailed plans about a weekend breakaway holiday than the arrival of a new member. Tell everyone, this is your baby's birthday, his only real birthday: it will never happen again. It is an occasion for all the family to celebrate. Of course, you may not want all the family around. That could be your idea of hell. If that's how you both feel, make sure your family understands that you want to be left alone; although it's always a good idea to have at least someone with you who is not so closely involved, preferably a friend or a member of the family who can be trusted not to fly off the handle if things go wrong at any time. Tempers can be frayed around this time.

Step 10: actualization

Forget everything you have ever read or heard about childbirth. Start from scratch. Enjoy the actual experience. Be there. Throw out all your preconceptions. Trust your intuition. Have the experience, not your thoughts about it.

Intelligent responses of the unborn child

There are other ways of communicating with the baby before birth and many researchers now believe it possible to give the baby what the Californian gynaecologist Rene Van de Carr calls a 'headstart' by various exercises that are said to induce intelligent responses in the unborn baby and help to develop his intellectual potential. Van de Carr is president of the Prenatal University in Hayward, California where parents are taught various ways of stimulating their unborn babies from the fifth month of gestation until birth. Van de Carr claims that the success of his methods is borne out by the large number of babies who are now entering kindergarten and first grade. 'Many of them,' he told a feature writer on the American magazine *Omni*, 'have attained high grades in reading and maths; they have highly developed social skills and they are confident as well.' ('Preschool?' *Omni*, August, 1989). I shall be describing the work of Van de Carr, and others who are carrying out research in prenatal stimulation, in the next chapter.

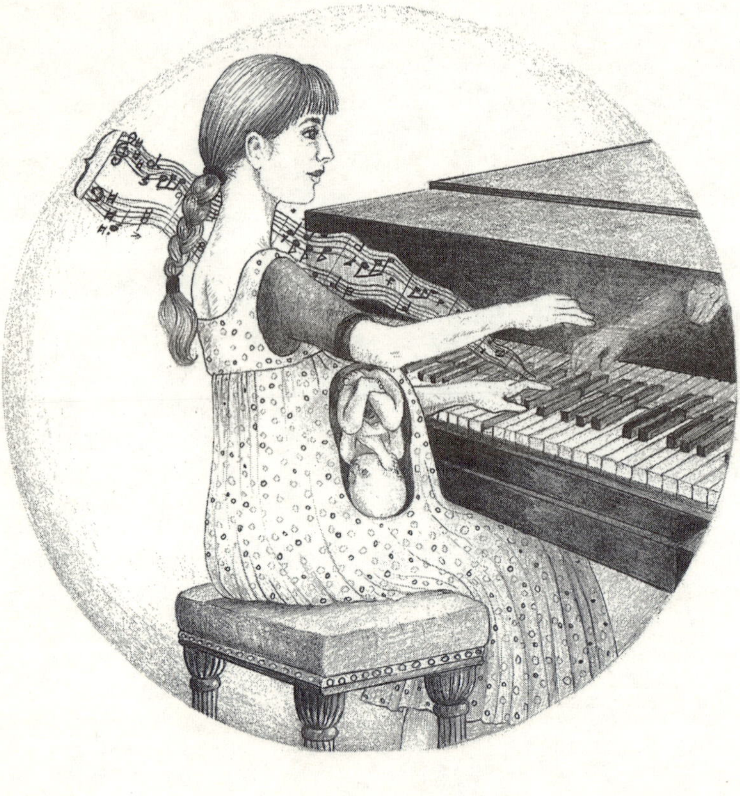

8

Prenatal learning

A six-year-old Los Angeles boy sits playing happily on the floor with his classmates. They are all singing an alphabet song. Two years ago, the little boy was deeply disturbed. A reporter on the *Wall Street Journal* describes how the boy used to throw hour-long tantrums (27 December, 1989). He would build a tower of bricks and then shout that it was on fire and knock it down in anger and terror.

His teachers were not surprised at his behaviour. They let him cry – it was a necessary release of tension – but they gave him lots of love. He had been completely neglected before and after birth. His mother was quite oblivious to the harm she was doing to him when she took drugs, including alcohol and cocaine, while he was developing in the womb. Then, after birth, she sometimes abandoned him in empty buildings. Once a building in which he had been left alone exploded in flames. So that's how he felt about buildings. They were lonely, inhospitable places that could burn you up. To him the womb must also have felt inhospitable, a poisonous place where there was no escape. No wonder the child cried and cried!

This child is one of a number who are taking part in a pilot study of children exposed to drugs in the womb. The children are not unintelligent – in fact, they seem quite normal in this respect – but they are considered at high risk for developmental, behavioural and learning problems. The long-term effects of maternal drug-taking during pregnancy are not known, but researchers believe that fine motor skills may be impaired and the children may have problems in forming attachments with others. The *Wall Street Journal* report describes the extremes of behaviour of these children, from apathy to aggression, passivity to hyperactivity, indiscriminate trust to extreme suspicion.

It is becoming obvious to many researchers that the rights of the unborn child are being widely abused, and no-one is doing very much about it. The drug users are obvious cases of people who are guilty of child abuse even before birth, but there are others less obvious. Care of the unborn child is an area that is grossly neglected. Mostly we concentrate on the health of the mother during pregnancy, and if the mother seems to be doing reasonably well in a physical sense. It is assumed that the unborn child will be developing satisfactorily. But this is not always the case. The child may be suffering while the mother carries on with a less-than-satisfactory lifestyle without doing herself any obvious harm in the short term. The unborn child's rights include the right to be loved and cared for from the moment of conception and the right to be protected from drugs, environmental pollutants, poor food, and not to be subjected to any kind of parental neglect. One researcher has gone so far as to compile a list of the rights of the unborn child (see box, page 121).

A social worker who is caring for the Los Angeles children says that they need lots of old-fashioned love. This is also true of the child in the womb. Of course, a couple who are deeply in love will want to do everything necessary to help their unborn child – their love child – to grow up in a healthy and caring environment right from the beginning of its life in the womb. Prenatal bonding depends on this love. But not everybody is aware of the many ways in which a child's development can be impaired, including his or her social and learning skills. Some get off lightly in spite of neglect; others become problem children. To counter any possible prenatal damage to the child's inherent skills a positive attitude towards the child must be adopted from the start of pregnancy.

There is plenty of evidence that this positive attitude has beneficial results later on. The Hayward gynaecologist Rene Van de Carr and his wife Kristin are two people who are dedicated to the care of the unborn child, teaching their mothers-to-be positive ways of bonding and nurturing the innate skills of their offspring. Their prenatal learning programme, as they call it, is attracting a great deal of attention in the USA; but more of this later.

The Fetal Bill of Rights

Drafted by Prenatal University, Hayward, California
February 24, 1989

The time has come to protect the rights of the as yet unborn child. Society's laws are meant to protect, not to harm, poison or kill. Every day, in every country throughout the world thousands and perhaps millions of unborn children are denied their natural right to normal development.

Prenatal University calls upon the concerned people, parents, educators and lawmakers of every nation to affirm once and for all the fundamental rights of the unborn child.

We hold these truths to be self evident:

That every unborn child has:

1. The right as a sentient being to have an unobstructed prenatal development.
2. The right to have adequate nutritional support to develop a healthy mind and body.
3. The right to be protected from exposure to poisons and toxins that retard neural and physical development.
4. The right to a healthy womb environment free of physical trauma or harmful levels of noise, light or other excessive stimulation.
5. The right to be accepted as an individual, alive and aware before birth.

If you believe as we do in the absolute necessity of establishing the above rights for your unborn child, the coming generations will respect and thank you for your courage and protection.

Let Every Child Become Your Own

By permission of Dr Rene Van de Carr and Dr Marc Lehrer

Prenatal research

Consider all the research that is going on in prenatal psychology and medicine, and also the experiences of a growing number of people who seek help for emotional problems from counsellors who include re-birthing in their therapy. You are bound to conclude that what happens in the womb is of crucial importance in the emotional and cognitive development of the child.

Research has shown that the autonomic nervous system of the premature baby is sensitive to the state of mind or the thought patterns of caretakers in his immediate vicinity. Either a relaxation or stress response can be induced in a premature baby by a caretaker's state of mind. Nurses looking after premature babies in intensive care wards say that they can significantly affect the health of infants through their attitudes. The premature baby has the same autonomic nervous system as the unborn child at the same gestational age. The only difference is that the premature baby is deprived of the mother's protection, which may tend to make him hypersensitive to stimuli. His reactions do, however, show how powerful thoughts can be in shaping the mind of a young life in its very early stage of development. The rejecting mother does produce a stress response in her unborn child; and the loving mother produces the relaxation response which is conducive to the development later on of social and cognitive skills.

Somatic basis of thought processes

In his fascinating book *The beginnings of Human Life* (Springer-Verlag, New York, 1977) the embryologist Erich Blechschmidt suggests that much of our thinking has its origin in the way we develop in the womb. In other words, physical processes initiated in the womb influence the way we perceive our world. They provide templates for our thinking and behaviour.

The development of the embryo at different closely linked stages has been carefully reconstructed by Blechschmidt in a unique collection in the Anatomical Institute at Göttingen University, which makes it possible to see every small change that takes place in embryonic development. What one sees is like a series of frames in a moving film. If you look at an individual frame it seems static, but it is just part of a continuous movement that is going on as the embryo develops. Each movement has its function. Each part of the body develops in a particular way, in unison with other parts, as a reaction to forces that impinge upon them from the environment. You can see the hand developing as a kind of grasping movement, while other parts of the body take up their positions – Blechschmidt describes them as 'positional movements' – with the movement of every part of the body related to what is happening in every other part.

Anything that impedes this natural movement can give rise to physical or mental problems in the child. Movement is life. The healthy body moves naturally in response to environmental stimuli, and this includes the way we think and behave. Our mental processes and our behaviour develop from the way we grow in the womb: from the way nerves develop and the way the growing embryo interacts with its environment.

Psychoanalysts led the way to an understanding of adult psycho-dynamics when they traced back some of our hang-ups, fears and inhibitions to early events, which were physical in nature, such as anal and oral fixations or the physical separation of mother and child or even perhaps, in some instances, the rejection of the mother's nipple by the child. Now it is believed that some of these problems can be traced back further still, to prenatal events. On the positive side, probably the way we pattern our world, the way we find pleasure in artistic creation, the way we think logically and search for answers to problems, are skills that developed from bodily processes: the way our nerves, our sense of touch, our hearing, our seeing developed in the 'good womb'. Our thinking, as Blechschmidt implies, developed as an extension of our body's sensory system. You can see this demonstrated most clearly in a child, much of whose thinking is closely related to its bodily needs and sensations, though there is a strong imaginative element present, arising out of a sense of wonder. Paediatrician Tom Bower, of Edinburgh University, has demonstrated that, contrary to what is commonly believed, children at a very early age are already capable of thinking in an abstract way, so this may well be a skill developed in the womb. Thinking develops as an essential function in a complex system of physical interactions.

If you are a scientist, you may find it difficult to accept the proposition that thinking is a kind of physical activity that is purely subjective, because you have learned to think in terms of a 'world out there' which is quite distinct from the world inside. But Blechschmidt has shown that even the most abstract mathematics has its foundations in bodily sensations and movements, initiated in the womb.

The hand is particularly associated with counting and measurement. Since earliest times the hand has been used for sign language; and it was out of this sign language, says Blechschmidt, that, over the centuries, we acquired the ability to systematize our thinking in abstract terms. But it was not until the sixteenth century that the functional development of the hand for scientific thinking became significant.

The main function of the hand is to grip things, enfolding an object with the fingers. And it was the fingers (digits) and the movement of the hands that formed the somatic bases of mathematics.

Blechschmidt describes the Arabic numerals, which were invented in the sixteenth century, as 'exact sketches of gestures of the freely movable hand when used as a tool'. The hands, which are used to hold, grip, grasp, etc. are object-bound. The mouth, which we associate with speech and sexual encounter (kissing), is person-bound. The two functions of hand and mouth may seem to be separate, but they are intimately connected with each other. The rooting reflex, which is a baby's instinctive searching for the mother's nipple, developed as the result of the movement of the hand towards the mouth in the early stages of development in the womb.

I give these examples to show how important different parts of the body are in the development of cognitive and behavioural skills. When we interfere with developmental processes in the womb in an unnatural way, we are in danger of damaging the child's mental functioning and behavioural skills. This is what happened with the Los Angeles children of drug users. On the other hand, if it is possible to stimulate developmental processes in a natural way, it may well result in an enhancement of cognitive and social skills. In fact there are those, like Dr Van de Carr, who say that we can do just that, and he claims many successes in prenatal stimulation.

Enriched environment

You can see the way learning develops as the result of physical stimulation in some experiments with rats. Berkeley University neuroanatomist Marion Diamond found in a series of experiments with rats, described in her book, *Enriching Heredity* (1988), that an enriched environment can change the brain and that rat pups of enriched mothers were superior at maze learning.

The brain is constantly changing in the womb and then during developmental phases after birth and even later as one grows older. The brain can be altered at any time of life: even in old age it has been shown to respond to stimulation, though it takes longer to produce any noticeable effect.

Marion Diamond's experiments show that the dimension of the cerebral cortex can be influenced through enriching the environment of both parents before pregnancy and enriching the female during pregnancy. 'The hypothesis we offer to explain these effects,' she says, 'is that the sex steroid hormones that are present at high levels in the mother during pregnancy might more readily cross the placenta barrier if the mother is a more physically active, enriched female, thereby "priming" the cortex of the developing fetus.'

Intrauterine education

This hypothesis is more or less the basis of Dr Rene Van de Carr's work at his surgery in Hayward, California. He has developed the concept of a teaching programme for unborn children. Over a period of time the programme has developed, expanded, and gradually evolved into what he now calls The Prenatal University.

The concept of intrauterine education is not new. It was practised in China over 2000 years ago. And even today in Japan, women practise an ancient technique of prenatal stimulation called Taikyo, which is believed to have beneficial effects on the baby after birth.

As long ago as 1970 Dr Van de Carr began to consider how a mother could make better contact with her baby before birth. 'My interest,' he says, 'was prompted by birth experiences which alerted me to different levels of consciousness of babies at birth.

Many mothers at the time were receiving large amounts of anaesthetics or medication as a matter of course. The relatively few mothers who used little or no anaesthetics were therefore of interest to me. Their babies appeared to be more alert and more "person-like."'

He then began to speculate about the implications of the heightened awareness and alertness of some babies at birth. He considered the possibility that the more alert babies had been more active and alert in the womb than was generally recognized at the time, at least during the last three months of pregnancy and that certain sensory capabilities had developed in them before birth. He also felt, in the case of the more alert babies, that the developing sensory system was being reinforced by the mother's own awareness of the child, resulting in an emotional interaction between mother and child.

In 1979 he began to develop his prenatal stimulation programme. It was a simple programme involving the parents in short sessions every day in which simple exercises were carried out. The programme was set out in a brief manual accompanied by a video giving examples of the exercises. Since then Dr Van de Carr has been joined by Dr Marc Lehrer and between them they have created a more comprehensive version of the programme which has proved a great success among thousands of parents who have been delighted by their ability to communicate with the unborn child.

Dr Van de Carr believes that obstetric care could be greatly improved in the United States and other countries by introducing his methods of prenatal stimulation. Besides helping the baby, these methods, he believes, have health benefits for the parents. 'I maintain,' he says, 'that this process has a tremendous potential for reducing complications during pregnancy, for reducing stress on the family during and after pregnancy, and for enhancing the health and the emotional and intellectual capabilities of the child.' He goes on to say (*Pre- and Peri-Natal Psychology*, Winter 1988) that parents who are considered at high risk for child abuse could be taught positive role behaviours before birth, rather than after the baby arrives and is making demands for attention. His programme has impressed a government department in at least one country. The Department for the Development of Human Intelligence in Venezuela has begun using his programme in rural and economically stressed areas in the hope of strengthening family bonding patterns, reducing child abuse and improving the intellectual capacities of children.

The programme

Parents who take part in the prenatal stimulation programme start communicating with the baby by using touch, vibration, motion, sound and light, which Dr Van de Carr claims the unborn child finds both pleasurable and stimulating. By about the fifth month a baby is capable of hearing voices, music and other sounds and feeling the pressure of physical contact via the surface of the abdomen.

The baby hears noises in the distance and feels vibrations and movement, but these don't reach him in any meaningful or patterned way. The parents' first goal, therefore, is to alert the baby to the fact that certain sounds and motions in the environment can have some meaning. The meaning is conveyed to the baby by the association of various sounds with the pleasure of being touched: for instance, by singing a lullaby while at the same time patting the abdomen in a rhythmical way.

At the beginning of the fifth month, a mother will begin to feel little kicks or movements in the lower abdomen. This is the time, says Van de Carr, to begin what he calls the 'Kick Game', which teaches the baby to respond to outside tactile and auditory stimuli.

The action of kicking, while the baby is moving buoyantly in the womb, is its way of exploring its environment. When a mother feels the baby kicking it is making contact with the sides of the womb. Dr Van de Carr's game helps the mother to give the baby the idea that its kicks can become a means of communication.

Dr Van de Carr says that the best time to carry out this exercise is between one and three hours after the mother has eaten, because the baby is utilizing the sugar from the meal and is at his most active and responsive. Either the father or mother can gently pat the part of the abdomen where the kicking occurs and, in the father's case, with the side of his head resting on the mother's abdomen, talk to the baby, asking him to kick again. This may sound a bit ridiculous and no doubt both parents will at first feel a bit cynical about the effectiveness of such a seemingly bizarre procedure, but it is a thrill for them when the baby does actually respond to the pats and talk. The talk must be baby talk: 'Mummy is talking to you. Kick Mummy again. Please kick Mummy again'; 'Daddy is here feeling your kicks. Do it once more. Kick Mummy again just here where I am patting you.' Of course the words will not be understood, but the child will pick up the sound of them and will associate particular sounds with the patting and kicking. Complete attention must be given to the child while this exercise is being carried out. It must feel as if the child is there before you, looking up to you for confirmation that you are there and that he is being cared for and loved. The closer you can get to this feeling, the more effective the exercise will be.

Lesson Two

Van de Carr describes the Kicking Game as lesson one in his prenatal learning class. Lesson two begins in the seventh month of pregnancy when the baby has reached a size where it is easier for parents to locate its head, back and bottom. (The diagrams on page 136 show you how to find the position of the baby). At this time the baby fits more tightly into the womb and is less mobile.

Two five-to-ten minute communication sessions per day are recommended, one in the morning when the mother will practise the exercises on her own, and the other in the evening when the father may also participate.

The mother is advised to lie on her back, but turned slightly so that her weight is on the left side, which will help to increase the blood flow to the womb.

Mother should speak at about three times normal volume, but try to avoid shouting or speaking unnaturally. Father should moisten his cheek with water (for better sound conduction) and should place that side of his face on the abdomen over the baby's ear and head. He should speak in a natural, reassuring voice as if expecting the baby to answer.

The exercises that follow make use of what Van de Carr calls primary words. These words will be accompanied by appropriate actions, such as rubbing, patting, squeezing. The idea is that the baby will be taught certain sounds that it will associate with pleasurable sensations. It is known that when a story is read to a baby at this stage of development he will recall the words (as sounds) later when the story is read to him after birth. This is the beginning of the learning process: prenatal communication makes the baby more responsive later to the sound of certain words. The parents' voices are also recognized by the baby after birth, and this is an important part of the bonding process. Music played to him regularly before birth will also be recalled after birth.

Examples of primary words are: *pat, rub, stroke, squeeze, shake, tap.*

The words should be spoken to the accompaniment of the appropriate action. You will pat the abdomen as you say *pat, pat, pat*; and rub the abdomen as you say *rub, rub, rub.*

The easiest part of the baby to locate is the back. It is a long, firm area at the side of the abdomen opposite to where the kicking occurred. The stroke exercise is done by placing your fingers over the baby's back near the bottom of the abdomen. Maintaining pressure on the back, move the hand gently upwards as you say *stroke, stroke, stroke.*

The squeeze exercise is done by applying pressure, gently but firmly, to opposite sides of the abdomen. And, as in the other exercises, say *squeeze, squeeze, squeeze.*

Shaking is done by placing the palm of the hand on one side of the abdomen and pushing in and out in a continuous, gentle, rhythmic movement and saying *shake, shake, shake.*

Tapping is done with one finger in a rapid motion against the baby's head, at the same time saying *tap, tap, tap* to the rhythm of the tapping.

Motion and vision

Dr Van de Carr's lesson continues with additional primary words in which the vestibular or motion sensors are used to teach words. These words have no tactile or touch components, but are associated with different qualities of sound or with visual stimulation.

For example, Dr Van de Carr suggests that the mother could stand on the bottom step of the stairs and let her heels slide off the stair so they come down sharply on the floor. When her heels touch the floor she will say loudly *drop.* Other words can be used to accompany different sounds, such as laughing, shouting, crying. When you sometimes become aware of a baby's spasmodic twitching which is believed to be associated with foetal hiccuping you could say *hiccup, hiccup, hiccup*. The word *music* could be used when you play music. Dr Van de Carr suggests placing a small cassette recorder on the right of the abdomen near the baby's head for this exercise, but he warns that the music should not be played too loudly: more than eighty decibels can disturb the baby. Whether the baby learns the word music or not, the sound of soft and soothing music is bound to be beneficial.

Mothers at Dr Van de Carr's clinic claim that in late pregnancy when they drink a lot of cold water, and say *cold* repeatedly, the baby often responds. The word *cold* should be said repeatedly about sixty seconds after you finish drinking. You can do the same after drinking hot fluids, saying *hot, hot, hot* after you have finished drinking.

Learn to talk to your baby, repeating words to describe whatever you are doing, such as climbing the stairs, washing, yawning, and so on. Involve your baby in all your activities. Tell the baby who you are: *This is mummy*. Encourage other members of the family to do the same: *This is daddy . . . this is John, George, Mary, Jane . . . this is Granny . . . this is Granddad*.

Dr Van de Carr suggests playing the same piece of music at the end of each exercise session. The same music should also be played intermittently during labour and at delivery. 'I am amazed,' says Van de Carr, 'at the apparent effect the music has on the baby during the birth experience.'

Visual stimulation is done by placing a very bright light in the lower part of the mother's abdomen in the direction the baby is looking. Then say the word *light* when the light is on, and *dark* when it is extinguished.

The effects of the programme

Dr Van de Carr claims that unborn babies who are stimulated in this way are given a head start in life. He has carried out tests on groups of infants who have participated in his pre-birth exercises, which, he says, show that those who had been strong programme participants spoke their first words earlier than moderate participants, and moderate participants spoke earlier than those who had not participated at all. He also says that some of his babies who have participated in the programme are now entering kindergarten and first grade. 'Many of them test in the ninety-ninth percentile for reading and maths,' he says. 'They have highly developed social skills and are confident as well.'

Dr Van de Carr's wife Kristin, a clinical psychologist, said in an interview (*Omni*, August 1989): 'We found that the mothers who started to connect with their kids in the uterus had a deeper knowledge of their babies. As a result the babies were easier to manage and the mothers were in a better frame of mind.'

However, there seems to be some disagreement between husband and wife about this. Dr Rene Van de Carr told me that as a result of his programme there could be what some might regard as negative effects. The babies who are stimulated in the womb are less likely to be passive, less likely to be compliant and are more interactive, they move more, and they may be more demanding and insistent on getting their own way. Not the sort of children mothers can manage very easily.

Not everyone agrees with Dr Van de Carr's claim that his programme has any effect on intelligence, though it is generally agreed that communicating with the unborn child can do no harm and can in fact help in creating a close family bond. My own feeling is that anything that creates a loving, caring atmosphere in the home, and recognizes the existence of another person in the womb and not just a medical condition called pregnancy, a person for whom both parents can feel responsible, is bound to lead to the sort of conditions that encourage learning and social skills. I don't believe that a child should be forced in any way, but the learning process should come naturally and spontaneously when the child is ready for it. As the Los Angeles teacher said of her disturbed children, the best way to treat a child is to give it lots of old-fashioned love. I prefer a child with a warm loving nature than one who is bright, but stubborn and difficult and wants his own way all the time. The intellect is not the most important thing in life. If the child thrives in a loving home, he will learn as much as he needs to know to live a happy, fulfilled life. I feel it is important that Van de Carr's exercises should be done in a loving and not an experimental way. This may well make all the difference to the outcome of the exercises.

I say that a child should not be forced, but what exactly 'forcing' is is another matter. Paediatrician Tom Bower believes that babies need much more stimulation than they have been permitted in the past; it is certainly not 'forcing' to play music or talk to a child in the womb, or to pat and rub him. It is feasible that a child who enjoys such an intimate and happy relationship with his parents from such an early stage of development will grow into a more socially skilful and brighter person than the average child, who is not regarded as there at all as a responding, wide-awake person until he is born, and may well have a higher than average IQ.

Baby tapes

The case for prelearning – the sensory enrichment of children before birth – has been put by Dr Brent Logan, director of the Prelearning Institute in Snohomish, Washington, who was mentioned in chapter 2. The unborn child who undergoes his stimulation programme, he says, arrives on the due date and gives his mother very little trouble. Labour is short and the child is born with his eyes wide open, smiling, his body relaxed, hands open, arms outstretched and no crying whatsoever. This is difficult to believe, but it describes the way a number of children entered the world and Dr Logan names them: Edward, Alice, Daniel, Natasha, Stephen, Martin, Burt, Janette and Brenda (identical twins) – all born since July, 1987, under a pilot study to evaluate prenatal stimulation.

Each mother in the study was required to play audiocassettes, of repeated sound patterns, which were placed on the maternal abdomen. The cassettes were played two hours a day, and changed weekly, for periods lasting one to seven months. The sounds were adapted from the maternal blood pulse, which is part of the unborn's sonic environment.

It has been known for about a century that a substantial number of brain cells (estimated at 75–90 per cent) in vertebrates die off shortly before or after birth. The excess cells that are discarded have been described as an 'overprogramming' to ensure that an adequate number survive to provide essential brain function. The process has been compared to the way the uterus is flooded with male sperm to ensure fertilization of the female egg.

Dr Logan's theory is that discarding so many brain cells is a terrible waste and if a few more were preserved at birth, the human brain would be much more efficient. Dr Logan's prenatal stimulation programme is designed to prevent the 'die-off' of so many cells and he says the results so far have been spectacular. Research into this method of prenatal stimulation is being carried out around the world with clinical trials in the USA, France, Germany, Japan and the Soviet Union.

The prenatal stimulation programme, known as the Cardiac Curriculum, starts with the normal sound of the mother's heart, with which the baby in the womb is familiar. Then the pattern of sound becomes more complex as the weeks pass, each week introducing a pattern just slightly more complex than the previous week's. Over several months each child hears up to 36 different variations of the cardiac-like sound, many more than normally experienced. In this way, as Dr Logan explains, the children are introduced to sequential learning based upon the primal rhythms of their environment.

The prelearning programme includes 16 audiocassettes called 'babytapes'. Any standard portable audiocassette player can be used and can be fitted into a comfortable fabric belt worn around the mother's abdomen. The pregnant woman starts playing the tapes at midterm (between weeks 20 and 24, the sixth month of pregnancy) although they may be introduced as late as the beginning of month eight. They are played at moderate volume for two hours daily, an hour in the morning or afternoon or evening. The kit, which is supplied by the makers, Prelearning Inc (16241 Cleveland Street, Redmond, WA 98052, USA) includes an instruction booklet and a journal to chart each baby's programme. The kit is available in the UK from Broadvale Associates, 17 Market Place, Brentford, Middlesex TW8 8EG (Tel: 081-568-7331).

Brent Logan says: 'Prelearners demonstrate consistent gains in intelligence, social skills and creativity – well beyond the norm. Unlike 'superbabies', these children show superior stress tolerance supporting sustained educational achievements.'

There are, however, criticisms of the programme from some professionals, the chief one being that parents' high expectations can do more harm than good. 'I do not think parents should want children to become little Beethovens or little Einsteins or whatever their idea of the perfect person is,' says

Dr Thomas Verny, author of *The Secret Life of the Unborn Child* (Sphere, 1982). 'Instead, we should use the window into the brain to tell the child that it is wanted and loved.'

New Jersey clinical psychologist Amy Altenhaus is also one of those who believe that the drive to have a brighter child, in the long run, does more harm than good. 'The pressure to be so exceptional,' she says, 'could turn the child into the equivalent of a burned-out broker on Wall Street by the first grade. There's so much to learn about the world. Why focus on reading percentiles of IQ?' (*Omni*, August, 1989).

The question is, what is intelligence? Is it about acquiring a high IQ and being good at passing examinations, or is it about being loving, caring, spontaneous, responsive, wide-awake and developing one's full potential as a human being? If it is the latter, as I believe it is, then prelearning programmes, which help to develop a child's natural abilities and full potential, should be encouraged.

Musical stimuli

I have mentioned a number of times the beneficial effects of music played to the unborn child. There is now evidence that the brain mechanism for musical development can be activated in the womb and there is at least one leading musician, Yehudi Menuhin, who attributes his musical talents to an exposure to music before and after birth.

Donald Shelter, Professor of Education at the University of Rochester's Eastman School of Music, is also one of those who believe that it is possible to develop musical talent before birth. He is in charge of a research programme which provides the unborn child with musical stimuli. Recorded music with a single melodic line is played to the unborn child through high fidelity stereo earphones placed directly on the mother's abdomen. For this purpose, Shelter uses orchestral music which is not too complex so that repeated patterns are absolutely clear. He believes that the baby uses the rhythmic and melodic pattern as a basis for further learning.

In 1988 he reported that thirty of his children who took part in his programme and were stimulated by music before birth visited him regularly for tests to evaluate their musical development. His tests included the measurement of attention span and body movements when music was played to them. Later he measured the child's ability to imitate rhythms and vocal sounds and to manipulate small sound-producing objects such as bells. Sessions in Shelter's music lab were videotaped for later analysis. He found that some of the children were able to imitate a two-or-three note melody within eight months of birth.

By the age of two, 80 per cent of the children were able to play the piano with one finger at a time rather than banging the keys in a random fashion as many small children do. The children sometimes play simple melodies and try them out at different places on the piano. They also sometimes sing the tune and there are some very bright children who will repeat the melody on other instruments.

The environment

One question that will be asked by some busy parents is: have we the time to devote to these prelearning programmes? They may both be going out to work until late in pregnancy. The answer is that most of the programmes are very simple and Brent Logan's baby tapes can be left to do their work while a mother is carrying on with her normal life. The programmes, however, will not work if there are other factors that interfere with the unborn child's development, such as environmental hazards and poor nutrition. The care of the unborn child must be total. The right kind of environment must be created and a natural, unharmful lifestyle must be followed by both parents if the child is to flourish and develop skills in the womb. The next chapter is concerned with these matters.

Finding the position of your baby

The baby's bottom feels soft, rounded and continuous with the legs. The part where you are kicked is usually high on the abdomen and opposite the bottom.

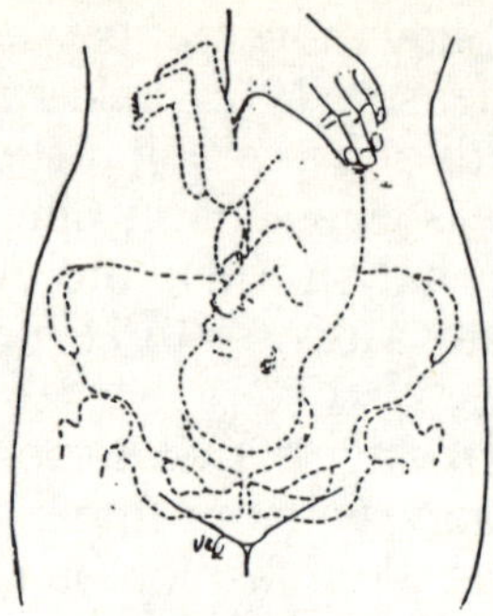

With one hand you can feel the firm smooth area of the back, while with the other you can feel the lumpy parts of arm and leg. You may find the baby to the side of the abdomen, more often to the left than to the right.

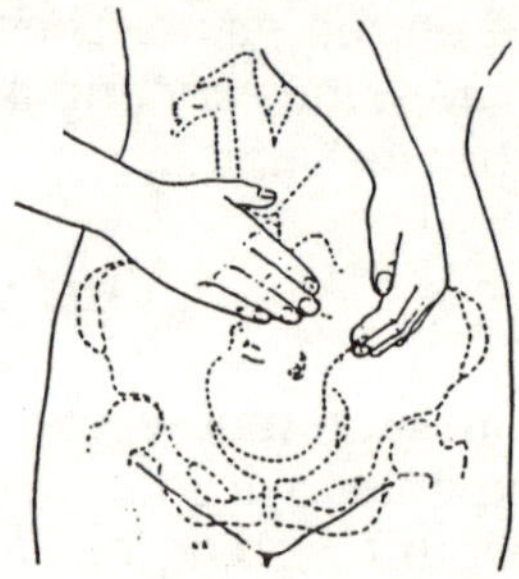

You can find the head just above your pubic hair. It will feel like a small round ball.

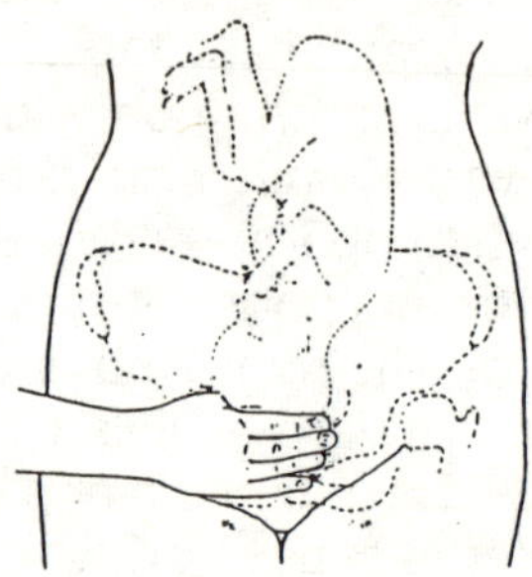

You can gently move the baby's head just a little way back and forth between the hands.

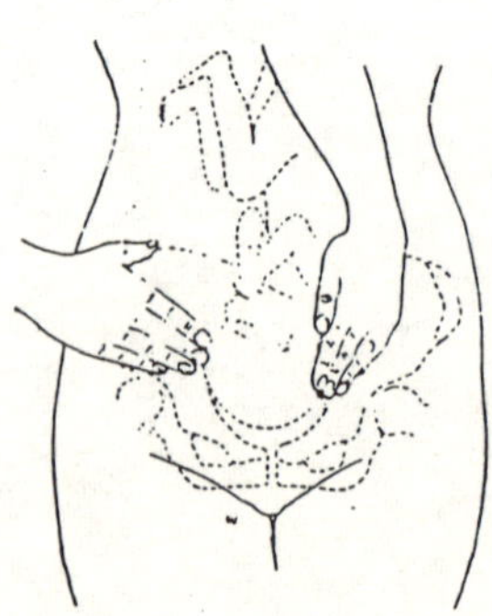

Adapted from Dr Van de Carr's prelearning manual (1)

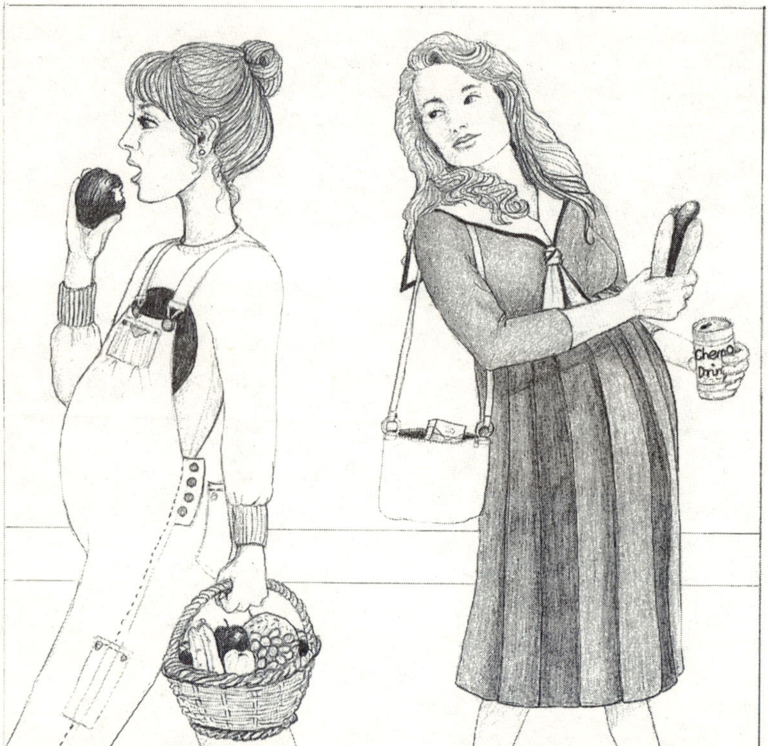

9

Cleaning up your neck of the woods

Most books on pregnancy devote a lot of space to the unpleasant things like morning sickness, tiredness, backache, and so on. It all seems so very painful and uncomfortable. It's important to know about these things, of course – about what to expect and how to avoid or alleviate pain – but too much emphasis is usually put on the medical aspects or the symptoms of pregnancy. This is because our culture regards health as nothing more than the absence of 'clinical symptoms'. The doctor's job is seen as mainly a matter of looking for what's wrong – i.e. for symptoms – and prescribing pills to suppress the symptoms. Our National Health Service is in fact misnamed. It's really a National Sickness Service.

Usually what doctors are treating are the normal workings of the body's defence mechanisms. These mechanisms – plus the well-established behaviour patterns that are inbred – have developed over millions of years of evolution to enable *homo sapiens* to survive the 'insults' of his environment – chemical, physical, infectious, psychological and social – and are essential for the maintenance of our health. For example, infected mucus which might be dangerous if it accumulated in the trachea is expelled by coughing. Similarly, toxic substances in the intestines are eliminated by diarrhoea. To interfere with these processes may give some relief by getting rid of the symptoms, but then other problems come along, the so-called side-effects of the pills and potions, which may in fact turn out to be a more severe form of the disease if the same medicine is given too often.

In any illness doctors should pay more attention to what nature is trying to accomplish. They should ask questions like

'What's right about the illness? What's good about it?' Not. 'What's wrong with the patient?' but 'What is the illness trying to do for the patient?' In fact, they should not be thinking in terms of illness at all for many common conditions, and certainly not in the case of the fairly common condition called pregnancy.

In Hippocratic medicine, even a crisis in an illness was seen as a point of growth. The emphasis was always put on the plus factor in any condition. In fact, the main job of the doctor was to be at the patient's side, to give him moral support, particularly during a crisis. The doctor didn't have to do anything very much. There was very little he could do anyway in a strictly scientific way. In fact, medicine down the centuries has always been more an art than a science. As Voltaire said, 'The art of medicine consists of amusing the patient while nature cures the disease.' It's never quite as simple as that, of course, but the doctor could, on occasions, do a lot more for his patients if he made them laugh instead of giving them pills.

The body – Dr Body, as someone called it – knows what to do. Throughout an illness the body is looking for ways of restoring its internal balance: i.e. the healthy and efficient functioning of all its parts, which should be working in harmony with one another. The body is always working: i.e. converting food into energy, throwing off infections, and so on. It is in a constant state of movement. And it is always moving towards stability, which is what the doctors call *homeostasis.*

In pregnancy we must work with the biological changes that are taking place in the body and not against them. Nature will see to it, in a healthy unpolluted environment, that the child will be cared for. Our job as parents is to make sure that the child is going to be born into a healthy environment. We can at least clean up our own neck of the woods. We must try to make our homes and workplaces free of environmental pollutants. It may take some doing – and you may have to make yourself unpopular campaigning for a smoke-free office, for instance – but this is certainly one of the best ways of ensuring the health of the child. By environment we mean everything around us on which we depend for our health, including food. It is important to know how your food is grown, where it is bought, and what chemicals in the way of preservatives or colourings or taste-enhancers are put into your food. We must be very careful these days, for the sake of the child, about the sort of food we eat and how we prepare it: hygiene is of the utmost importance.

Doing what comes naturally

If you look at a pregnant woman from a non-industrialized African or South American community, you will still see her going about her ordinary, everyday tasks, and you will be struck by her poise and her ability to get on with things in a matter-of-fact way, without much fuss. There is no suggestion of illness or of anything abnormal about her condition. She is simply going to have a baby. That's all – and, of course, that's enough! It's the baby who is important. It may seem the most obvious thing to say, but it must be said all the same that to this woman the baby growing in the womb is what is making her look the way she is, not the fact that she is suffering from some kind of medical condition, which is the way Westerners often see the expectant mother. She is simply 'growing big with child'. That was the biblical description of pregnancy. But many people, particularly men, either show no interest or avert their eyes. They don't see a child there at all. They just see the pregnant woman carrying all that weight and suffering the consequences.

For the woman from a non-industrialized society, pregnancy is something that happens very frequently, which she knows how to handle perfectly well. For the baby to be healthy, the mother merely has to go on being herself, living a healthy outdoor life and eating healthy food. (This, of course, is not true of some Third World countries nowadays, but it is still true of many people who continue to live simple lives, miles away from civilization – for instance, tribes who still live in the depths of the South American rain forests.)

The pregnant woman in such a community has the support of her tribe and all the womenfolk in her extended family. Birth is very much a family event. This closeness of the family helps the bonding process. A place is prepared for the child: he's expected; he's wanted; he's loved. This makes for a trouble-free pregnancy, without any of the stresses and strains we know in the Western world.

The gist of what I am saying is that looking after your baby is a matter of staying healthy yourself or of preventing yourself from becoming unhealthy, in mind and body. Unfortunately, most of us do not live simple, straightforward lives, close to nature. In fact, we tend to live incredibly complicated lives, nowhere near nature, and are governed mainly by two principles: (1) 'the pleasure principle'; and (2) a driving force, dating from the Industrial Revolution, which the Victorians called 'the work ethic'. Neither of these principles is of any use to anyone really. They do more harm than good. The trouble is, we have separated work from play, and made one the reward for the other: pleasure as reward for pain. In a sense, life is all work. There's nothing particularly virtuous about work. Work – the stretching of muscles – and play – the rest and relaxation that comes afterwards – should not be regarded as separate activities. The separation of work and play is not so obvious in non-industrialized societies. Even some of their dances and rituals are connected with work: they are performed to appease the gods so that the rains come, or the sun shines, and the harvest is gathered; and their work is rewarded with food and shelter, not with money or property, or things to own. When you're close to nature, you hardly notice what's going on in your body or your way of living, because it's all going on as it should do in a natural way. You are part of earth's eco-system, and, as such, no one has to tell you what to do. You know it in your bones.

Largely because of our post-Industrial Revolution lifestyle, we are threatened by all kinds of health hazards in the environment – at work, in the home, in the streets, in crowded public places. There are poisons in the food we eat and in the very air we breathe. So staying healthy is not so easy these days and it's not getting any easier.

In present-day circumstances how can expectant parents bring about conditions that will give their child the best possible start in life? Can anything be done to protect the child, who is already threatened in the womb by pollutants that get into the mother's body and cross the placenta? And what are the known teratogenic agents (i.e. harmful to the growing embryo and foetus) in food? We shall leave others to advise parents on the purely medical aspects of keeping fit during pregnancy (there are many books on the subject) and concentrate on what for many is the main enemy today, which is the environment. Get that right and you'll find you have an easier time during pregnancy and childbirth, and your baby when he arrives will be healthier.

In the following pages we point out some of the main environmental and food problems and how they can, to a large extent, be overcome.

Health hazards in the environment

Lead

One of the main pollutants of our towns and cities is lead, a poisonous metal that has been in use for thousands of years. No doubt it has been responsible for a lot of illnesses in the past (it has been suggested that the madness of some Roman emperors may have been due to the high lead content in all the wine they drank), but it is only recently that we have become aware of what damage it can do, particularly to the central nervous system in its early stages of development.

High lead levels can cross the placenta and damage the growing embryo and foetus. There is evidence that it damages the bones and liver and it can induce miscarriages. It also has a deleterious effect on mental development and capability, and behaviour after birth. The deleterious effects begin at conception and continue throughout prenatal development.

People living near or on main thoroughfares and children in school playgrounds near traffic are exposed to high levels of lead. This is mainly because of lead in petrol. There's lead in the dust in playgrounds; in foodstuffs sold at open stalls in main roads; in flaking paint or the dust from this; in the unlined seams of food cans; and in some tap water where lead piping is still in use or where copper piping joints, which contain lead alloys, are used.

If you live in an old house, the chances are that there is still some lead piping. If this is the case, water from the tap should be allowed to flow for some time before using. When you are re-decorating, make sure you wear a mask when scraping off old paint or sweeping a room afterwards. If you are living on a main road, keep your front windows shut during the rush hours or when traffic is heavy, and sleep and eat in the back rooms. It's best not to live on a main road if you can help it. Don't eat vegetables that have been bought at an open stall without washing them thoroughly first.

You can be tested for lead levels by hair analysis. If you are pregnant, lead levels should not exceed 1-2 ppm (parts per million). If levels are high, it may be possible to lower them through Vitamin C supplements combined with certain trace minerals.

Cadmium

Cadmium has a long biological half-life (i.e. the time it takes to reduce the metal by half through decay) and consequently it tends to accumulate in the organs, especially the kidneys. Prolonged exposure to cadmium can be extremely damaging to the kidneys.

Levels of cadmium build up in the placenta and foetal tissue and block the transport of other essential minerals. Cadmium and lead together, apart from poisoning the child, prevent the uptake of zinc, a trace element which is required for a wide range of cellular activities, many of them vital for growth and development. It has been found that women who smoke tend to have high levels of cadmium. This is another reason why a couple shouldn't smoke during pregnancy. And remember, other people's smoke can be harmful, so keep to non-smoking areas in restaurants and other public places.

Mercury

Doctors have tended to play down the possibility of mercury poisoning, except in very unusual circumstances, because the body can absorb quite high levels of the trace metal without ill-effect – as much as 2 milligrams a day. But what the medical profession has been unaware of until quite recently is that quite low levels of mercury in the mother can be damaging to the unborn child. The reason for this is the 'mercury trap'. The unborn child traps the mercury selectively and it accumulates in the foetal brain.

There was a famous case in which pregnant women were poisoned by mercury when, following an accident at a plastics plant in Japan, alkyl (including methyl) mercury was released into Menamata Bay, poisoning all the fish there. The fish were eaten in large quantities by families in the area, and it was found that children subsequently born to women pregnant at the time were physically or mentally deformed, although, much to everyone's surprise, the mothers were not affected. The level of mercury in foetal blood was about 28 times higher than in the mothers' blood.

You should therefore be very careful not to absorb even the smallest quantity of mercury during pregnancy, and this includes some dental amalgam which contains mercury. A woman should either insist on fillings which don't contain mercury, or avoid fillings around the time she is likely to conceive and throughout pregnancy. Your water supply should also be checked for mercury.

Aluminium

It has long been thought that aluminium was a poisonous substance and it has been linked to cancer of the stomach, though there is no evidence for this; but now scientists are beginning to have their suspicions and one study pointed to the possible association of aluminium in tap water and Alzheimer's disease.

In view of the uncertainty about the toxicity of aluminium, it would be wise for the pregnant women to avoid using cooking utensils made of aluminium and to test tap water for the presence of the metal, which is used by some water boards for purification purposes. Some medicines prescribed for indigestion contain aluminium and should be avoided.

Copper

Although in small quantities copper is an essential trace element, it can be toxic in large quantities. Lead can raise tissue copper levels, and high levels of copper, like most heavy metals, can interfere with the activity of many enzymes. Copper is believed to be one of the contributory causes of lead encephalopathy, a serious disorder of the brain. There may be copper in areas where the drinking water is soft and acid.

Health hazards in the home

When you are making plans for your baby's arrival, you will want to make sure that your home is free of anything that could damage his health. Among the main health and safety hazards are:

Electricity

Make sure that your wiring is safe. Have it checked now. Faulty wiring is a frequent cause of fires. Also make sure there are no open plugs into which little fingers can fit and no dangling wires attached to electric kettles, irons etc. Wires trailing across the floor could be dangerous when you are pregnant.

Microwave ovens

These generate electro-magnetic radiation (microwaves) and could be harmful to the unborn child. Some of the old types of ovens are leaky. Check that yours is not one of these. The modern types are subjected to stringent safety tests by official 'watchdog' organizations – in Britain, the British Electrotechnical Approvals Board – and are regarded as safe, but there are a number of basic precautions covered in the instruction leaflet. Always read the instruction leaflets issued with electrical appliances.

Electric blankets

Never plug an electric blanket into an adaptor in which another appliance is plugged, or in a light fitting. Check your blanket regularly for signs of wear – e.g. scorch marks, frayed edges, damaged flexible cord. You should get an expert to check your blanket at least every two years.

Water

Get your water checked if you suspect pollutants. The main pollutants, which vary from place to place, are lead, nitrate, aluminium, iron and manganese. In Britain, lead is a problem in soft and acid water areas, such as north-west England and Scotland. In hard water areas it is rarely a problem. But in all areas it can be a problem where plumbers use a lot of lead solder in the joints of copper pipes. There are also thousands of old homes which still have lead piping. Nitrates are of concern to more than 900,000 consumers in Britain, supplied by 52 water supply zones in Lincolnshire, Norfolk, Cambridgeshire, Staffordshire and other areas of Yorkshire, Anglian and Severn Trent Water Authority Regions.

Water filters

The answer to water pollution may be a water filter, but not all of those on the market are effective against all pollutants; and some may even increase the pollution in your tap water. The

Thames Water Authority has found bacteria as much as 1000 times higher in some filtered water than in the tap water. Most jug filters and many plumbed-in cartridge filters contain activated carbon which removes chlorine and temporary hardness; it also reduces levels of certain heavy metals, including lead.

There are some filters that contain a resin which removes nitrates. If there is enough resin in the cartridge, this can be a very effective way of reducing nitrate levels. For a list of reputable water filter manufacturers see resource section at the end of the book.

Pets

Although dogs and cats can be wonderful companions, they can be a source of infection and, if you don't already have a pet, it would be wise to postpone acquiring one until the family is well established. Keep all pet dishes scrupulously clean and away from your own dishes. Don't encourage pets to lick you.

Hygiene in the home

In these days of food poisoning reaching epidemic proportions, hygiene is more important than ever before in the home. Some of the bugs that get into food have been around a long time and are very common. Our own skin plays host to a remarkable number of bacteria. At any one time there can be as many as three million on one square centimetre of your skin. That is why it is so important to wash your hands thoroughly before handling food. And, of course, any sores or cuts on hands should be dressed. Make sure your kitchen is always spotlessly clean and that there is adequate, efficient storage space for food. Lavatories, of course, are a high risk area in terms of bacteria. The lavatory seat and lid, cistern, handle, and door knob or handle should be regularly wiped with a clean, damp cloth and disinfectant. The lavatory bowl should be frequently treated with disinfectant left overnight in the water before flushing away. See also *Main Reasons for Food Poisoning*, page 153.

First aid

Always keep a first aid kit in the home as well as in the car. The kit should contain:

- A mild liquid antiseptic such as TCP, Dettol or iodine.
- A clinical thermometer.
- One packet of waterproof adhesive plasters of different sizes.
- Sterile prepared dressings, which consist of pads attached to varying lengths of bandages and are quick and easy to put on.
- Triangular bandages to make slings or secure dressings.
- Two gauze (open weave) bandages and several crepe bandages.
- One large packet of cotton wool.
- Calamine lotion, for soothing burns, stings, etc.
- Tweezers (blunt ended), scissors, safety pins.
- Bottle of aspirin or paracetamol or gentler analgesics (herbal or homeopathic).

It would also be advisable to add a few emergency items needed for a baby such as remedies for colic or fever. Choose non-toxic herbal or homeopathic remedies. Nelson's Pharmacy in London produce a homeopathic first aid kit consisting of six tablets and three creams for emergencies. For the address see resource section at the end of the book.

Health hazards at work

We are just beginning to realize how much damage some chemicals in common use, such as various petroleum products, are doing to our environment and our health. Manufacturers of these chemicals have been telling us for years that they do no harm, but clinical ecologists keep finding allergic illnesses and teratogenic effects (i.e. harmful to the unborn child) caused by many of these chemicals. The list is a long one and is still growing. They include petrol and petroleum products, paints and glues, pesticides, combustion products from cars and burners, dry cleaning fluids, chemicals used in photocopying machines, fluids used for cleaning carpets, plastic and foams. The golden rule is *if you can smell it, suspect it.* This, however, is not foolproof. There are poisonous chemicals that have no smell: but they may announce their presence by symptoms such as a headache, watery eyes, a runny nose or a skin rash. If you are working with a chemical and you develop any of these symptoms, consult a doctor, preferably a clinical ecologist and, if she confirms your fears, enlist her help in getting a transfer to another job.

VDUs

There is believed to be a link between VDU usage and miscarriage/birth abnormality. It is not, however, established whether the trouble lies in ionising radiation, which is known to produce birth defects and miscarriages, or the stress of working for long hours in front of a VDU screen and the bad posture of many operators.

As a sensible precaution, if you are expecting a baby, it would be wise to avoid working with VDUs. If this is not possible, then you should not work for longer than four hours a day with a VDU. Make sure that your posture is right when sitting in front of a VDU and that the design and layout of the workstation minimizes visual and postural stress. Make sure that the VDU screen is shielded against glare and static electricity.

Muscular problems and repetitive strain injuries

There are a number of conditions from which sedentary office workers, who spend long hours in repetitive jobs, suffer. They include upper and lower backache, pain in legs and ankles, assorted muscular strains, sore neck and shoulders, and repetitive strain injuries. Most of the problems are caused by a combination of uncomfortable postures and sitting for long hours working with a VDU without regular breaks for rest and relaxation away from the workstation. These conditions of work are quite unsuitable for a pregnant woman, who could suffer some injury that could incapacitate her and make it difficult to do quite simple tasks for a baby. For example, tenosynovitis, or Teno, the most common of the repetitive strain injuries, in which the tendons of the wrist and fingers are injured, can be quite serious and make it difficult for a woman to lift anything: lifting a baby could be a problem. Repetitive strain injuries can also afflict factory workers who do repetitive jobs with their hands. The problem in all cases is the over-use of muscles; and the solution is to relax and exercise the muscles at regular intervals and not to work for long hours at any particular job.

Food fit for your unborn baby

It's very worrying for anyone nowadays to know if the food in the shops, particularly convenience food, is really fit for consumption. Where indeed, you may well ask, is it safe to buy any food? Even the most reputable supermarkets have been guilty of selling contaminated food. However, not all convenience foods are junk. Frozen peas, for instance, have more vitamins in them than fresh peas. But there are so many foods, such as poultry, eggs, soft cheeses, salami and other pre-cooked chilled products that are suspect and can poison you and your child. Quite apart from the danger of contamination somewhere along the food chain, the food we eat is not really very good for us anyway: for years now many of us have been eating all the wrong foods. Those of us who have been advocating health foods, and have been dismissed as eccentrics, have been proved right.

It is only just beginning to dawn on our critics that much of the food that we eat, even food we once regarded as healthy and essential for the pregnant woman, such as eggs and milk, is of very poor or indifferent quality. And the main reason for this is the popularity of certain types of convenience foods that we call junk food (that are mostly lacking in essential nutrients) and the widespread use of chemical fertilizers and pesticides combined with present-day farming practices, where animals are kept under unnatural conditions and wrongly fed. All the poisons in the soil and in the atmosphere are producing what one writer called 'the poisoned womb'.

There have been a few wise nutritionists who, for years now, have been warning us about the dangers of eating too much of the wrong kinds of food and not eating enough foods that are rich in natural fluids, in fibrous bulk, vitamins, and minerals, and not too rich in calories. This is the sort of diet that was advocated by that famous Swiss dietitician Dr M. O. Bircher-Benner, the inventor of muesli. Over fifty years ago he was saying things that only now have become accepted by dieticians. His main contributions to diet, apart from muesli, were his recipes which consist of raw foods and the use of vegetable protein-fat milk (soya milk) as a substitute for cow's milk. He introduced us to the delights of natural food. Raw vegetable salads (in which raw turnips and cauliflower can be used with more traditional salad vegetables) go down very well with a yoghurt dressing (yoghurt, lemon juice, some onion and dried green herbs) or mayonnaise without eggs and made of a mixture of soya flour (or milk), oil, lemon and water.

Bircher-Benner also insisted that you should start the day with something raw to eat – some fruit or vegetables – food that does not lie too heavily on the stomach but which keeps us satisfied for long periods and cuts out the need for mid-morning snacks.

What we have discovered in recent years is that a healthy diet can also be a very enjoyable one; and furthermore it keeps us alert and energetic between meals. This association of a good taste, a feeling of satisfaction after a meal, a clear head and a body that is working well is what a balanced diet aims to achieve for you. There are quite a number of cookbooks nowadays that give numerous mouth-watering recipes for meals that satisfy without putting on weight, and even some books for people who have to follow special diets (e.g. for diabetics) that can be used by everyone, because they cut out much of the sugar and fat that make people ill.

Eating for a healthy baby means eating well yourself and choosing food that is good and enjoyable for all the family. However, there's a slight difference. Because the pregnant woman is having to increase her body's load of work, she will have to eat a little more of certain foods, particularly foods that are rich in vitamin C, folic acid and some other vitamins and minerals (see tables on page 157-59), and she won't be able to indulge herself so often in the way she did before she was pregnant: she could get away with it then, but not now! It is believed that some of the minor illnesses of pregnancy, such as morning sickness, may be aggravated if not caused by the wrong sort of diet.

The important thing is to treat yourself to a wide variety of nourishing foods which provide you with all the essential nutrients: protein, carbohydrate, vitamins, minerals, etc. Individual needs vary, depending on size, age, height, the sort of work you do, and so on, and the pregnant woman will most likely know what her own needs are better than anyone else. If you cut out junk food and food high in sugar and fat, you will know what is good for you and your unborn child. You need not worry too much about weight now, while you're pregnant, so long as you have no medical problems, such as diabetes, and are not grossly obese: then you will need expert medical attention. But for most pregnant women this is not the time to start slimming. You can postpone your weight-reducing programme until after the child is born.

Eating without risk

You will, if you are pregnant, probably be worried about reports of infection getting into a lot of food, and you may be afraid that all the food you enjoy most is just the sort of food that can make you and your child ill, or lead to complications at birth or even to the death of your child. Such things do happen nowadays, and sadly, with increasing frequency.

So what can you do about it? The Bircher-Benner diet is the right one for you if you are fed up with supermarket convenience foods (where some of the problems arise), and you want to get back to a more natural way of eating that is good for you and your baby: this is a way of eating that is likely to be without risk. The old way of buying food, from the butcher, the baker, the grocer – in other words, from someone you know very well whom you can trust, is the best way. But there are very few of these individual shops left, alas!

Maybe the risk of catching some awful disease by eating pre-cooked food is not very high, but for the sake of your baby, you will not want to put yourself at any kind of risk at all.

Although pregnancy is a perfectly healthy condition, the expectant mother must make sure that her diet will help the growth of her baby and will provide her with the energy to cope with all the changes that take place in her body, without overtaxing or depleting her strength.

She will also need the kind of nutrition to combat the common symptoms of early pregnancy, such as early morning sickness and abnormal cravings.

The sort of directions given by Bircher-Benner dieticians are:

1. Follow your natural instinct, which is usually the right guide to the choice of foods that are good for you in your condition.
2. Make sure that you get all the nutrients you need so that your body can cope with the extra workload, but don't think

you must 'eat for two'. Your body's way of dealing with food is to utilize everything it receives with economy and efficiency.

3. The Bircher-Benner rules should be adhered to strictly. These are: fresh food as a start to every meal, two or three raw vegetables daily, as many green leaf salads as possible, wholemeal cereals, no high-fat junk food or any food in packets or cans, no pre-cooked and pre-chilled food, no pastry cooked with white flour, no stimulants, such as coffee, tea or alcohol. Only a little salt should be used; a herb seasoning makes a good substitute.

If you stick to these principles you will find life a lot easier during pregnancy. Tables 2 and 3, devised by Jill Metcalfe for diabetics (but suitable for all pregnant women) will help you to plan recipes that provide you with all the nutrients you need. If you are not diabetic, you might like to add some other foods, such as molasses (a rich source of iron), honey or butter; other varieties of cheese such as Cheddar; and full cream milk. But go easy: too much sugar or fat is no good for anyone. A hard Dutch cheese, which is low in fat, is preferable to some soft cheeses that are low in fat, and have always been recommended for diabetics, but which nowadays may be suspected of carrying listeria.

Main causes of food poisoning

- Food prepared long before consumption and not refrigerated
- Cooling food too slowly before refrigeration
- Use of already contaminated cooked food
- Not reheating cooked food at sufficiently high temperature
- Undercooking
- Not completely thawing frozen poultry before cooking
- Cooked food stored close to raw food resulting in cross-contamination
- Preparing food on contaminated surfaces
- Contaminated dishes
- Cleaning dishes with dirty dishcloths
- Dishes washed in same water as pet bowls
- Hot food stored below 63 °C
- Infected food handlers
- Use of leftovers.

Nutrient	*Uses*
Vitamin C Needs are virtually doubled during pregnancy	Important in the production and maintenance of healthy tissue and the production of your and your baby's increasing blood supply. Vitamin C ensures the body absorbs enough iron from food and so makes a healthy supply of blood.
Vitamin A Needs don't really increase until you are breastfeeding, but as Vitamin A can be short in many diets, extra attention to the good sources during pregnancy is important.	Needed to ensure proper formation of the hair, nails etc, maintenance of good vision, and helps protect against infection.
B vitamins in general The need for all B vitamins goes up slightly during pregnancy and breast-feeding.	Needed to help control digestion and the use of nutrients (including energy) from the food we eat. Shortages will lead to the poor development of the baby.
Folic acid A member of the vitamin B group, the need for which increases by at least two-thirds during pregnancy.	Failure to have enough folic acid will mean that the baby's new tissue and blood supply will not form properly. This is a vital nutrient – make sure you are getting enough.

Nutrient	*Uses*
Vitamin D Normally exposure to sunlight is enough to provide all the vitamin D we need. But during pregnancy take care to ensure you are getting enough, by going out in the sun and eating foods that are rich in vitamin D.	Vital in the absorption of calcium to make strong teeth and bones. Calcium needs more than double during pregnancy and breastfeeding so extra vitamin D is essential. The body does store some vitamin D, so providing you have previously had lots of sun and you are topping it up with regular exposure during the pregnancy plus eating some rich sources of vitamin D, extra supplements should not be necessary.
Calcium The need for calcium increases dramatically to more than double that of the non-pregnant requirement.	If your diet is lacking calcium the new teeth and bones that the baby is forming will not be strong and calcium will be taken from your bones, leading to problems later in life.
Iron Iron intake increases a little due to the need for an increased blood supply.	Sufficient iron is essential to form haemoglobin, which is the oxygen carrier in the blood. This oxygen is essential for the growing baby and to maintain the health of the placenta.

Nutrient	*Uses*
Protein and calories Both of these increase slightly during pregnancy, but most diets provide more than enough protein. Most mothers get a bigger appetite which more than compensates for the extra calories they need. For many it is a case of eating normally rather than consciously cutting down.	Small increases required to cover the extra work of forming the baby, maintaining the placenta and carrying the extra weight.

Food	Good sources	Amount to aim at	Use
Cheese – medium fat	Excellent source of calcium and protein and some B vitamins. Watch amount of fat though.	**2-4oz (50-100g) week**	For sandwiches, flavouring sauces, in flans or with soups etc.
Cheese – low fat e.g. Edam	Good source of calcium and protein and some B vitamins	**4oz (100g) or more week**	As spreads or in cooked dishes
Milk – semi skimmed	Excellent source of calcium, protein and some B vitamins	**At least 6 pts (3 litres) per week**	In drinks, on cereals, in savoury sauces, puddings etc.
Milk – evaporated	Good source of vitamin D (as often enriched) and calcium. Some B vitamins	**2-4fl oz (50-100ml) week**	Use to make porridge, enrich custards and sauces. To accompany fruit puddings or in cooked desserts
Eggs	Source of some iron, B vitamins, vitamin A and a little vitamin D	**5 a week**	As a main meal, snack or in sweet or savoury dishes
Margarine	Enriched with vitamins A & D. Watch quantities because of fat content	**Max 4oz (100g) week**	For baking etc.
Low fat spreads	Enriched with vitamins A & D. Some brands also contain a little calcium. A good choice for those who are watching their fat intake	**Max 4-6oz (100-150g) week**	For spreading, in sauces and in some baking

Food	Good sources	Amount to aim at	Use
Breakfast cereals	Buy high fibre or wholegrain versions wherever possible for extra fibre. Good source of B vitamins and of some iron because enriched	**1oz (25g) or more day**	Breakfast, mid-meal snack or bed-time snack. Use as a base with stewed fruit etc.
Wholemeal/granary bread/rolls or wholemeal pitta breads	Source of B vitamins, some iron and folic acid	**25-40 slices week. Equivalent to 2lbs (1 kilo) bread or bread products**	For sandwiches and snacks, with main meals, soup etc.
Liver – all types	Good source of iron, folic acid, vitamin A and B vitamins	**5-6oz (125-150g) week**	Grilled, casseroled, or made into a pate or spread
Meats (red) e.g. beef, pork, lamb, mince etc.	Source of iron, protein and some B vitamins	**2-3 helpings (4oz (100g) raw weight) week**	Extend with vegetables, especially pulses, but when using cheaper cuts trim or skim off any visible fat
White fish and poultry if properly defrosted and well-cooked	Good source of protein	**3-6oz (75-150g) week**	Use instead of red meats once or twice a week. Roasted, sautéd, stir fried, grilled, baked or casseroled
Mackerel or kippers	Excellent source of vitamin D and some vitamin A and calcium and protein. Also contains all essential fats	**4oz (100g) week fresh smoked or tinned**	Grill or bake as a main meal or made into a spread for use in sandwiches, dips etc.
Tuna or pilchards	Excellent source of vitamin D and some calcium. Choose those in brine or tomato sauce	**2-4oz (50-100g) week**	Use as main course with vegetables, pasta, rice, etc. or as a filling for sandwiches

Food	Good sources	Amount to aim at	Use
Fresh/frozen vegetables or salad	Good source of vitamin C if cooked quickly or eaten raw. Green leaf vegetables contain useful amounts of Folic Acid and vitamin A. Strongly coloured vegetables such as peppers, carrots, swede, sweet corn are a good source of vitamin A	**At least 1 large helping of 1 or more vegetables or salad every day**	With main meals, to extend meat and poultry dishes, as a meal in themselves when eaten with added egg/cheese/pulses/nuts. Try to have some raw vegetables e.g. carrots, tomatoes etc. at least once or twice a week
Peas, beans, lentils i.e. pulses	Source of iron and protein and some B vitamins. An excellent source of dietary fibre	**At least 2 helpings a week. Either 1oz (25g) of dried beans or 4oz (100g) cooked or tinned beans for each helping**	Use in soups, casseroles with meat, poultry or vegetables or mixed with fish or liver for a spread in sandwiches
Vitamin C rich fruits e.g. oranges, tangerines, grapefruits, guavas, blackcurrants, blackberries etc.	Excellent source of vitamin C and some vitamin A	**At least 1 helping a day of 1 or a combination of fruits from this group**	Eat fresh on their own or as an accompaniment to breakfast cereal, dessert etc.
Fruit e.g. apples, pears, bananas, etc.	Good source of vitamin C	**At least 1 helping day**	Eat fresh on their own or as an accompaniment to breakfast cereal, dessert etc.
Fruit – dried	Source of some iron and vitamin A – especially dried apricots	**Once or twice week 1oz (25g) portion**	Mix with breakfast cereal or in cooked items

Reprinted from February 1987 *Balance*, The Magazine of the British Diabetic Association, 10 Queen Anne Street, London W1M 0BD.

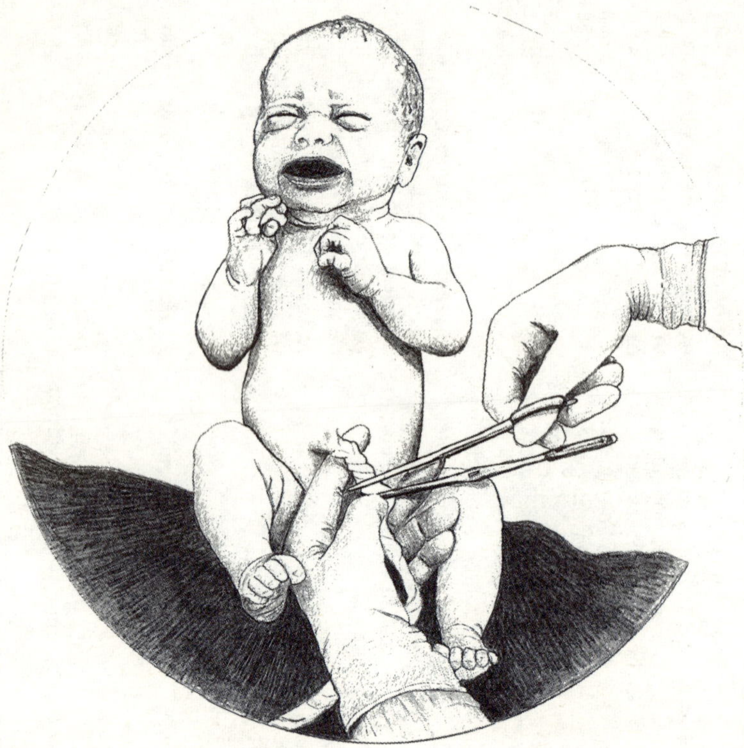

10

Cutting the cord — ending a relationship

'Cutting the umbilical cord' are powerful words. They arouse all kinds of feelings, like cutting a lifeline, depriving you of sustenance. It happened to you. The scar, which we call the belly button, is still there. The cord is in fact something that is never completely lost: it's always there in the memory. Before the cord was cut you were a different being. You were more spiritual. You were one with the universe. One with everything. No inside and outside, no good and bad: the Buddhist state of Nirvana. Then suddenly you're split off; and it seems as if for the rest of your life you are trying to become whole again. Is this a schizophrenic fantasy? Or is it the reality? Isn't this the sort of thing that goes on happening all the time – losing something and then regaining it; never quite losing anything – a recurring pattern in our lives?

'Man knows the universe in the womb. He forgets it at birth', said the Jewish mystic Martin Buber. He was referring to what he called the I-Thou relationship, which was the unity of a mother and child before the child became aware of himself as a separate person. In other words before there was an 'I' or ego. At the beginning the child had no sense of being a separate person. That experience in the womb or in early childhood comes back to us sometimes as a 'peak experience'. It is a moment of bliss that has a special quality which is difficult to describe. Freud called it the 'oceanic' feeling.

A sense of oneness is felt throughout the early years of infancy. You are where you are and what you are doing. The memory of this feeling inspired Wordsworth to write of 'intimations of immortality' from recollections of early childhood, and the British metaphysical poet Henry Vaughan to write:

I cannot reach it; and my striving eye
Dazzles at it, as at eternity.

The modern playwright Eugene Ionesco is referring to the same feeling when he writes about his 'desperate nostalgia for paradise'. Paradise was the bliss of being in the womb.

The cutting of the umbilical cord brings to an end the sense of oneness of the I-Thou relationship; and then a separate self, the 'I' without the 'Thou', begins to develop, very slowly at first. It is some time before 'shades of the prison house' as Wordsworth described the developing awareness of the hell that is the 'ego', begins to close in on the growing child. It need not be hell, but for many it is. The child is afraid of his sense of separateness. When danger threatens he runs to his mother: he sees his strength in that unity of mother and child. Without her he is nothing. The unity he sensed in the womb had a quality that stays with him all his life; and that quality can shape his whole lifestyle. He either had what some psychologists call the 'good womb' experience or its opposite, the 'bad womb' experience, or something in between. At an early stage of development a mother's love and respect for her child will seem to the child no different from self-love and self-respect, which is the perfect bond. It is mainly a physical sensation of being bathed in love (the good womb) and this will lay the foundation of a loving, caring nature, respecting the needs of others as well as oneself. A mother's rejection or neglect of her child, in or out of the womb, will result in 'disbonding' and create a self-rejecting, self-destructive personality.

The psychoanalyst Otto Rank was the first to talk of 'the trauma of birth'. That, in fact, was the title of a book he wrote in 1929. In substance, his theory is that separation from the mother at birth produces feelings of anxiety that are often reactivated later in life as a result of a threatened or actual separation from someone or something. The most obvious separation occurs when someone you love walks away. Then a memory stirs in you and you start feeling anxious . . . Will he fall under a bus? Will his plane crash? Will he be killed on the motorway? 'In every parting there is an image of death', said George Eliot. That image of death, according to Rank, is a memory of birth. It felt like death when you came to the end of your life in the womb. It was the first of those life events that can be so disturbing . . . first day at school, first day in a new job, suddenly being thrown out of work, bereavement . . .

Rank said that it was very common for patients with some mental illness to have fantasies of returning to the womb. If the patient is psychotic, no help can be given, says Rank – 'he loses his way in the labyrinth of the womb'. If, on the other hand, he is mildly neurotic or disturbed 'he finds his way back to health . . . by threads of remembrance thrown to him by the analyst.'

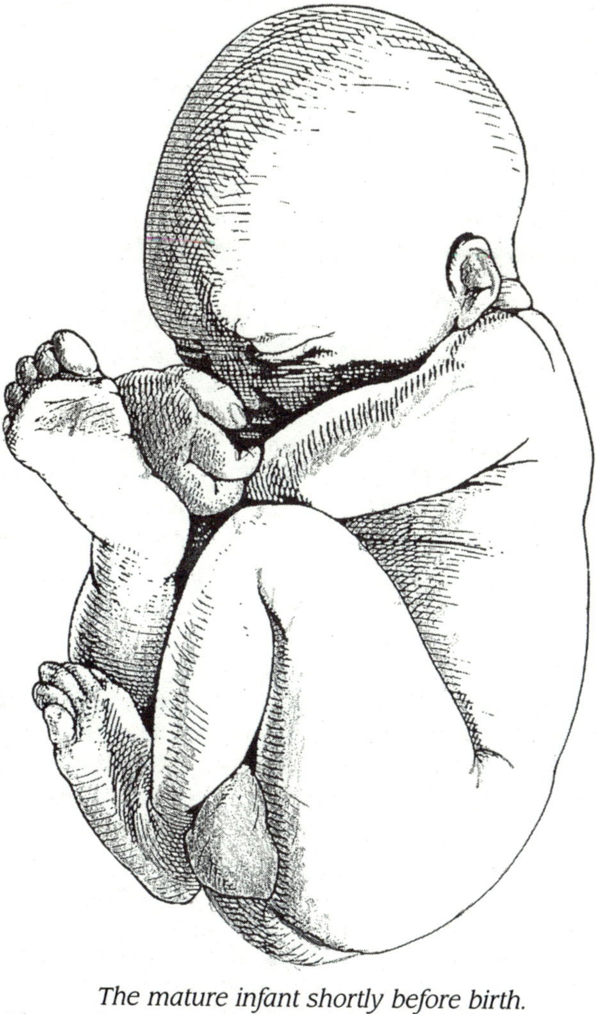

The mature infant shortly before birth.
From *The Beginnings of Human Life* by Erich Blechschmidt (1977)

Dr David Winnicott, a paediatrician and psychoanalyst who practised just before and after the Second World War, was also interested in birth trauma. In working with his patients he believed in the principle of non-interference and would allow patients, children or adults, to manifest physically their 'body memories' of birth experience.

Writing of a middle-aged woman patient who had had several years of classical analysis, without any effect, and was suicidal, Winnicott said that 'she must make a very severe regression'. He also said that he would 'follow the regression tendency wherever it led'. Winnicott went on:

> In the patient's previous analysis there had been incidents in which the patient had thrown herself off the couch in an hysterical way . . . Eventually I recognised how this patient's unconscious need to live the birth process underlay what had previously been an hysterical falling off the couch.

Winnicott described how, when the patient did relive the birth process, every detail of it was retained: 'not only that, but the details had been retained in the exact sequence of the original experience'. The patient acted out the sucking of the thumb in the womb, the constriction passing down the birth passage, the pressure on the head and also 'the extreme awfulness of the release of pressure on the head, during which phase, unless her head was held, she could not have endured the re-enactment'. When the regression reached what Winnicott called 'the limit of the patient's need', there was a natural progression, 'with the true self instead of a false self in action'.

Winnicott, however, did not regard the normal birth as a traumatic experience. Birth, he said, was, of course, a separation – 'a break in the continuity of the infant's going on being' – but trauma only occurred, in his view, if there were a severe disturbance at birth which prevented ego development.

Rank suggested that the trauma of birth could well be necessary for the survival of the child. Without it, the child would regress to a state of immobility and unresponsiveness to verbal communication, which is what the catatonic does. The child must be 'anchored in anxiety'. Those moments in later life – the so-called life events when there are dramatic changes of circumstance – reactivate the feelings of anxiety that kept the child alive. Rank described these feelings as a 'therapeutic intervention by nature'. It is like the anxiety you feel when crossing a busy road – a normal anxiety – which keeps you alert and on your guard, and gets the adrenalin flowing. Not an unpleasant experience. So there's nothing wrong with the anxiety of birth: for most, nowadays, it is perfectly all right. But for some, anxiety becomes trauma.

Birth for the baby

Since Winnicott's day there have been thousands of re-enactments of births, through the various re-birthing techniques already described. Dr David Chamberlain wrote about some of these re-enactments or memories of birth in an article called 'Babies Remember Pain' published in the *Journal of Pre- and Perinatal Psychology* (Autumn 1989). From all these memories Dr Chamberlain is able to say something about the way a baby finds the world when he arrives and he asks various questions. 'Babies are famous for their cries at birth', he says. 'Is crying normal? Some babies make no cry and instead gaze at their parents with total concentration. Have they no complaints?'

The answer, for most babies, is that they have a lot to complain about. When they cry they are often in pain; and the cry is a cry of protest. Dr Chamberlain describes why newborn babies cry:

> They cry when they arrive in a delivery room that is twenty degrees colder than they were used to in the womb. They cry when they are being wiped and washed and being stretched out and measured. They complain when given injections (vitamin K) and eye drops (antibacterial). They react to skin puncture. Crying rates and heart rates shoot up as heels are lanced for blood samples.

One of Dr Chamberlain's patients remembered, under hypnosis, an early experience in his nursery when he was sick:

> I'm bothered by the nurse. She keeps coming in, taking my temperature, taking blood. I wish she would just leave me alone. The other thing that was annoying was the shot. That was more pain . . . I see the nurse leaning over me. She has a shot with

> something in it. She took the cap off it and checked it for air bubbles. She rubbed my left arm with alcohol and gave me a shot. It hurt! And I wasn't prepared for it. Then I became very tense and screamed. It really bothered me and I cried a long time after that.

One of Dr Chamberlain's conclusions, after studying many reports of the pains suffered by newborn babies, was that despite mounting evidence of infant pain, the characteristic reaction of medical practitioners was one of denial.

What I have been trying to demonstrate in this book is the three-fold nature of caring for the unborn child. 'Holistic' medicine approaches pregnancy in this way, looking first at the psychological or spiritual aspects of the way a twosome, a man and woman, becomes a threesome, mother, father and child; secondly at the physical aspects – biological and genetic; and thirdly, the environmental influences, including the food we grow and eat, the way we tend our cattle, all the ways in which we produce food, and other environmental influences – the material things (cars, buildings, cities etc.) chemical (e.g. poisonous waste from industry), the political and the social. The three aspects cannot be separated. All three are related and all impinge on what happens to the child. The most important time in his development, governing to a large extent the way he adapts to the environment in later life, is the time he spends in the womb.

Birth for the mother

If both parents have carried out all the exercises suggested in this book, the birth should be what Leboyer described as 'a gentle one'. But nothing can be guaranteed and – I'm sorry for repeating this – perfection is unattainable. Someone once said, 'if it's not surprising, it's not true'. So something surprising will probably happen to you – and the odds are for you it will be a pleasant surprise. Anyway, I hope so. Whatever happens, it will be *your* experience – so enjoy it, or at least learn something from it.

Coping with labour

No one can say just how a woman will handle her labour. It is an experience that is bound up with the character and lifestyle of the expectant mother. And she herself will not be able to say with any certainty how she will cope. But the various exercises you have done regularly, and the sessions of planning you've spent with your partner, will certainly help you through the experience and you may well find that the pain is not so bad as you expected. No one, however, can promise that there will be no pain. Not enough importance is attached to pain in antenatal classes; in fact most advice is a bit negative, building up fear in the woman. She fears the worst; and that fear in itself can bring about a resistance that will make the pain worse that it need be.

The pain of childbirth is the pain of *opening up,* literally and metaphorically, involving the mind and heart as well as the body. A big part of the pain, of course, is the physical stretching of the cervix and vagina, but it has a different quality to it than just physical pain. It is more like an expansive energy flow than a pain. A powerful force which takes you over. The pain is resisting this energy flow, a resistance which for most mothers is both mental and physical. The way to deal with the pain is to stop resisting it, if you possibly can, and to go along with what is happening. If the effort is too much, there are, of course, various chemical ways of easing the pain – and no one will blame you if you call for one of these. Gas and air is the least harmful. It takes the edge off contractions. The advantage is that there will be no ill-effects afterwards for you or your baby.

But a positive attitude to the experience, going along with it all the way, a determination to enjoy it, and the emotional support of a partner, relative or friend, will lessen the pain or at least make it more acceptable.

'I was in tears from start to finish of my labour', said one mother, quoted in the magazine *Practical Parenting.* 'Not from pain; I could cope with that. It was just the emotion. The very best experience of my life.'

Birth position

A lot has been said about the advantages of an upright birth. There are important psychological benefits. The Brazilian doctors Moyses and Claudio Paciornik, who made a film about the squatting position, said:

> In the *supine* position the *before* and *after* stand out as intense moments, while the moment of birth dilutes itself because of the diminishing of the active maternal participation which is unstructured.
>
> In contrast, the squatting position allows a transition which links the *before* and *after* birth. The uninterrupted exchange of stimuli facilitates the emotional rapport between mother and child, especially her confidence in mothering. A baby born this way is thus stimulated by human love rather than artificial procedures.

Lying prone is offering yourself to the obstetrician or midwife. The squatting position, on the other hand, gives you the feeling it's just you and the baby, with the emotional support of your partner, who are involved. It is more a part of the bonding process and less confusing to the child whose whole thrust is downwards.

Elizabeth Noble, director of the Maternal and Child Health Center, Cambridge, Massachusetts, points out that if knowledge was all that birthing women needed, then the 'experts' would have the easiest births – and that is rarely the case. She believes that the unfolding of labour depends on intuitive knowing, faith in the wisdom of the body and trust in the natural process of birth-life-death. She is against the experts giving instructions like Push, Push, Push – which make the mother feel inadequate – and leaving everything to the mother's intuitive knowledge of what to do.

Birth for the father

It's much more fun being a father nowadays. When Dorothea and I had our first child I was sent home after I'd accompanied Dorothea in the ambulance to the vegetarian nursing home, which was supposed to be a progressive place, but was quite old-fashioned compared to the normal labour ward today. I was told I wasn't wanted. I'd only be in the way, they said. And Michael, my eldest son, was born only half an hour later while I was making my weary way back home across London in bus and Tube. I'd been looking forward to the birth of our baby, but I accepted what everybody told me that this was woman's work and it was best for me to stay out of the way.

Things are different now, of course. But there are still some fathers who don't know what's hit them when the baby arrives. They know that they can, if they wish, be present at the birth: but some of them regard that as a bit of a chore, if not an imposition: they'd much rather be going to work or waiting outside in a pub. They are all churned up, of course, though they dare not admit it. Their attitude is the old-fashioned one of take it on the chin! Or something of the sort. A positively Victorian attitude which still lingers: the masculine stiff upper lip!

I don't know how many of that type of father are around today, but I'm sure there are still a few. Only the other day I heard a young man, whose wife had just produced a baby (which he'd reluctantly agreed to) saying how he'd done his duty – and that was that! He had no idea what was ahead of him except that it was going to be pretty awful – sleepless nights and so on! He thought of himself as a martyr in the cause of babyhood.

I liked the young man. And I wondered, was he just turning the whole thing into a bit of a joke because underneath he was scared? Did he really believe what he was saying? And it occurred to me that you can get very heavy about all sorts of things in life, and at just those times when you should be on top form and enjoying yourself hugely, all the fun goes out of life. And if there's one time when you should retain your sense of humour it's when a baby arrives. The whole ritual – the long faces, the frenzied activity after the waters break – can really be terribly funny if you are able to stand on one side and just look at yourself.

So, remember, father, keep smiling! A father's role hasn't changed much over the years. He's there mostly to give emotional back-up to his partner – and a sense of humour is a great help. The father we have been writing about in this book has been more involved in pregnancy and childbirth than most fathers, so he will feel more able to cope when labour begins. He knows that there's nothing really to worry about although many mums do worry that they might not know they are in the first stage of labour and may not make it to the hospital in time. Of course, mums do know they are in labour by the time it's established and their cervix starts opening. And the new dad, who has been monitoring the growth of his child in the womb and has been almost as close to him as his partner, will not panic when the time comes to go to hospital or to call the midwife.

No one, however, can say when labour will begin. It can start at any time within two weeks of the estimated date of birth. So, if you're going to have the baby in hospital, make sure the two of you have a suitcase ready containing all the essential things you will need. A father should make himself responsible for preparations of this kind. He should also act as spokesperson for his partner in asking questions and seeing that she gets all the care and attention in hospital that she has every right to expect, and is not bullied by obstetricians or nursing staff. His job is also to keep visitors in order or at bay after the baby arrives, and to see that his partner is not bothered by a string of cooing relatives around her bed when she and the baby need some sleep.

There is not much more to say except that research has shown that the father who has been involved in the pregnancy from the very start and has had some antenatal training is far better able to cope with looking after the baby, changing nappies and so on, than the father who has had no training. And it has also been found that the baby benefits enormously from the co-operation of both parents in looking after him and remaining close to him. Emotionally he is more stable than a child whose father remains at a distance. So to both of you, I wish you a happy time, and I know you are going to have the happiest and healthiest baby you can possibly have, if you go along with the suggestions I've made in this book. But – for the last time! – don't expect perfection. You'll have your share of problems, that's for sure. Just be what Bettelheim described as good enough parents!

Useful addresses

Active Birth Movement, 32 Cholmeley Crescent, Highgate, London N6 5JR.

ASH (Action on Smoking and Health), 5-11 Mortimer Street, London W1N 7RH. Tel: 071-637 9843.

Association for Improvements in Maternity Services (AIMS), 163 Liverpool Road, London N1 0RF.

Association for Spina Bifida and Hydrocephalus, 22 Upper Woburn Place, London WC1H 0EP. Tel: 071-388 1382.

British Diabetic Association, 10 Queen Anne Street, London W1M 0BD. Tel: 071-323 1531. BDA produce a Pregnancy Pack, including the *Pregnancy Network,* a list of women who would be happy to have other diabetic women contact them.

Cystic Fibrosis Research Trust, Alexandra House, 5 Blyth Road, Bromley, Kent BR1 3RS. Tel: 081-464 7211.

Foresight (The Association for the Promotion of Preconceptual Care), The Old Vicarage, Church Lane, Witley, Godalming, Surrey GU8 5PN. Tel: Wormley (042879) 4500. They publish *Guidelines for Future Parents.*

Haemophilia Society, 123 Westminster Bridge Road, London SE1 7HR.

Health Education Authority, Hamilton House, Mabledon Place, London WC1H 9TX. Tel: 071-631 0930. They publish a leaflet called *So you want to stop smoking.*

Herpes Association, c/o Spare Rib Ltd., 27 Clerkenwell Close, London EC1.

Holistic Rebirthing Institute, 184 Lansdowne Drive, London E8 4NE. Tel: 071-267 8739. (Information provided by Judith Collingon).

Institute of Optimum Nutrition, 5 Jerdan Place, London SW6 1BE. Tel: 071-385 7984.

Maternity Alliance, 15 Britannia Street, London WC1X 9JP. Tel: 071-837 1265. Campaigns for improvements in rights and services for mothers, fathers and babies.

Meet a Mum Association, 26a Cumnor Hill, Oxford OX2 9HA.

National Childbirth Trust (Education for Parenthood), 9 Queensborough Terrace, London W2 3TB. Tel: 071-221 3833.

Parent Network, 44-46 Caversham Road, London NW5 2DS. Tel: 071-485 8535. Brings parents together to share their experience of family life and learn from each other.

Pre-Eclamptic Toxaemia Society (PETS), Dawn James, 88 Plumberow, Lee Chapel North, Basildon, Essex SS15 5LP.

Pregnancy Sickness — for telephone counselling, 0943 609 209 or 0851 5016.

Relaxation for Living, 29 Burwood Park Road, Walton-on-Thames, Surrey KY12 5LH. Tel: (0932) 227 826. Supply relaxation tapes and cassettes.

Society of Teachers of the Alexander Technique, 10 London House, 266 Fulham Road, London SW10 9EL. Tel: 071-351 0828.

University of Surrey, Stag Hill, Guildford, Surrey GU2 5XH. Tel: (0483) 571281. They hold two-day workshops on integrative regression (rebirthing) based on the style of Frank Lake and William Emerson.

VDU Workers' Rights Campaign, City Centre, 32-35 Featherstone Street, London EC1. Tel: 071-608 1388.

West London Birth Centre, 7 Waldemar Avenue, Ealing, London W13. Will provide addresses and information concerning local birth centres. Send stamped, addressed envelope.

Yoga for Health Foundation, Ickwell Bury, Northill, Bedfordshire.

Infant Developmental Education Association, UCLA Medical Center, Factor 5-942, Los Angeles, CA 90024, USA.

Maternal and Child Health Center, 2464 Mass Avenue, Cambridge, MA 02140, USA.

Pre- and Perinatal Psychology Association of North America, 13 Summit Terrace, Dobbs' Ferry, NY 10522, USA.

Prelearning Institute, 2000 Lake Street, Snohomish, WA 98290, USA. Tel: (206) 568 3329

Prenatal University, Calaroga Clinic, 27255 Calaroga Avenue, Hayward, CA 94545, USA

International Society for Prenatal and Perinatal Psychology and Medicine, Engelbrektsgatan 19, S-11432 Stockholm, Sweden.

Index